8 Weeks to

Women's Wellness

The Detoxification Plan for Breast Cancer, Endometriosis, Infertility and Other Women's Health Conditions

Dr. Marianne Marchese

About the Author

Marianne Marchese, ND is a clinician, author, and educator. She graduated from Creighton University with a Bachelor of Science in Occupational Therapy in 1990. Dr. Marchese received her Doctorate of Naturopathic Medicine from the National College of Naturopathic Medicine (NCNM) in Portland, Oregon. She completed a two-year postgraduate residency in Integrative Medicine and Women's Health and completed a six-month post-graduate training in Environmental Medicine.

Dr. Marchese has been an adjunct faculty member at the National College of Naturopathic Medicine, Life Chiropractic College, and currently, she teaches Gynecology at the Southwest College of Naturopathic Medicine in Tempe, AZ.

Dr. Marchese is a highly sought after speaker and has presented at seminars and conferences throughout the U.S. and Canada. She has had articles published in numerous magazines and journals and currently writes a bi-monthly column on environmental medicine in *The Townsend Letter*.

Dr. Marchese maintains a private practice in Phoenix, AZ and was named as one of *Phoenix* Magazines' Top Doctors for 2010. *8 Weeks to Women's Wellness: The Detoxification Plan for Breast Cancer, Endometriosis, Infertility, and other Women's Health Conditions* is Dr. Marchese's first book.

Learn more at *www.drmarchese.com*

8 Weeks to
Women's Wellness

Dr. Marianne Marchese

SmartPublications™

PO Box 4667
Petaluma, CA 94955
www.smart-publications.com

613.04244 MAR

Published in the United States of America

First Edition, 2011

Library of Congress Control Number: 2011920481

ISBN: 0-9843635-5-6   978-0-9843635-5-1

Warning—Disclaimer

Smart Publications™ has designed this book to provide information in regard to the subject matter covered. It is sold with the understanding that the publisher and the author are not liable for the misconception or misuse of the information provided. Every effort has been to make this book as complete and as accurate as possible. The purpose of this book is to educate and entertain. The author and Smart Publications™ shall have neither liability nor responsibility to any person or entity with respect to any loss, damage caused, or alleged to have been caused, directly or indirectly, by the information contained in this book.

"Smart Publications" is a trademark of Morgenthaler Family Limited Partnership, a Nevada Limited partnership.

TABLE OF CONTENTS

ACKNOWLEDGMENTS

This book has been years in the making and would not have been possible without the help and support of a few key people in my life. Thank you to Mary Beth Ryan-Maher, Dr. Lise Alschuler, Kathleen Feeney, Dr. Lyn Patrick, Dr. Joni Olehausen, Chris Tomasino, Bill Gotlieb, Dr. Dan Carter, Brendan Mahoney, Dr. Kimberly Windstar-Hamlin, Dr. Jane Guiltinan, Dr. Peter D'Adamo, Dr. Chris Meletis, and Kate Williams.

Thank you to everyone at Smart Publications and Health Freedom Nutrition for working hard to make this project come to life, especially John Morgenthaler, Dale Fowkes, Ed Kinon, and Neal Ratchford.

To Dr. Walter J Crinnion for whose willingness to share his vast knowledge and experience I am so grateful. He is truly the 'father' of naturopathic environmental medicine.

I especially want to acknowledge my mentor, colleague, and friend, Dr. Tori Hudson. She taught me everything I know about being a naturopathic physician and, specifically, women's health. She embodies the principle of 'doctor as teacher' and continues to work tirelessly to pass onto others her extensive knowledge of women's health.

A very special thank you goes to my mother and father for all of their love and support over the years. I will never forget the night I was living in Chicago and my father called me from Omaha to say he had just watched a TV show about alternative medicine. He told me it was going to be the medicine of the future, and that I was making the right decision to go back to school to become a naturopathic physician. He said, "Marianne, work hard and have tunnel vision—tunnel vision."

Finally, to Margie; thank you for putting up with years of "doctor talk" and for all the love, encouragement and support that you have provided. I am so grateful that God put you in my life. I am truly blessed.

FOREWORD

Dr. Marchese does a wonderful job in *8 Weeks to Women's Wellness* to present vitally important information which will help women regain and retain their health and vitality. The unfortunate fact is that we are all carrying a body burden of chemical toxins that we acquire, first from our time inside of mom, and then from the air, food and water we intake. This burden is growing greater with each year and each new generation, and is associated with many serious health problems. Many of the health problems that are caused by these compounds are generally thought of as consequences of aging. But, in reality, the majority of these problems are from the addition of more toxins to our body, rather than adding more years to our age.

Dr. Marchese reviews the classic avenues of toxin exposure so that the reader can more easily avoid building up their burden. Since having a body full of toxins ends up costing all of us a lot of money (medical bills and the cost of cleansing), it makes perfect sense to avoid, as much as possible, contributing to that toxin load. With the information that Dr. Marchese provides on how these exposures occur, it becomes much easier to keep our load from building. She goes on to review the specific health problems that have been linked to toxic burden in the medical and scientific literature. While many people typically only associate cancers, such as breast and ovarian cancers, to pesticide exposure, a great many other health problems are toxin related, as well.

The classic presentations of toxin overload include fatigue, "brain fog", fibromyalgia, thyroid problems, depression and chemical sensitivity (any adverse physical, mental or emotional symptoms after breathing a chemical fume). But many women can experience a host of other illnesses that are toxin-related including: infertility, endometriosis, uterine fibroids, miscarriage, osteoporosis and polycystic ovarian syndrome. By reviewing this section in *8 Weeks to Women's Wellness*, many women will finally be given the answer to their questions of "Why am I ill?", and more importantly, "What can I do about it?".

But, Dr. Marchese doesn't stop there. She then takes the reader on a journey of discovery and healing. Discovering the types of toxins that are in one's body and reviewing the currently available tests for these compounds is vitally important to begin the healing process. It is very important to note here that the standard allopathic physicians, as wonderful as they are, do not receive ANY TRAINING in this area. In fact, the training that is available in the area of toxicity is based upon industrial hygiene standards (i.e. What is the level of workplace toxins that can be in the blood without the person being incapacitated?). So, you may want to buy an extra copy of *8 Weeks to Women's Wellness* to give to your favorite allopathic physician! She or he may end up learning a lot of valuable information.

The healing journey is then presented by Dr. Marchese and includes detailed information on how to best avoid the greatest sources of toxin exposure that we all have (primarily our indoor air and the food that we eat). She then presents steps to take to REDUCE the burden of toxins that we carry. The importance of this for young women who are preparing to become pregnant cannot be over-emphasized. Please give copies of this book to all the young women you know who want to have the healthiest children possible. You will be doing them a huge favor, as Dr. Marchese has done for all of us by providing this important and extremely helpful book.

Walter J. Crinnion, ND

Department Chair Environmental Medicine, Southwest College of Naturopathic Medicine.

INTRODUCTION

Is there a link between chemicals in the environment and women's health conditions? A woman's body is dominated by monthly hormonal changes involving estrogen, progesterone, and testosterone. Maintaining a balance of these and other hormones is vital to women's health. Conditions such as breast cancer, fibroids, endometriosis, PCOS, miscarriage, and infertility are all influenced by hormones. Chemicals in the environment can affect a women's reproductive system.[1] Over the past half century, the production and use of man-made chemicals into our environment has increased. It is no coincidence that during this same period, disease and illness in women has also increased. The fact is that most of the chemicals developed in the U.S. have not been tested to determine if they can harm human health and influence women's hormones.[1]

Recently, the medical community has started to focus on the link between chemicals (toxins) in the environment and health. When I first started medical school, I didn't know anything about environmental medicine, which is the study of the interaction between chemicals in the environment and human health. Thankfully, the school I attended offered a course in environmental medicine. Also, the medical clinic where I trained had a supervising physician who saw patients with health conditions linked to chemical exposure.

But it was during my post-graduate residency with Dr. Tori Hudson that I unknowingly took that first step toward becoming a leader in environmental medicine.

In general, our health care system is set up to treat the sick, and not prevent the sickness. If you have some strange symptom and go to the doctor, your blood will be drawn, studies performed, medications given or surgery offered. If your symptom goes away, then you are cured and considered a success of the system. If your symptoms continue, eventually you will be told nothing is wrong, and you'll be sent to a psychiatrist and placed on antidepressants. Typically no one asks why you have this symptom, or what its cause may be.

My career in health care started in the late 1980s while I was an undergraduate at Creighton University. I entered occupational therapy school, intent on helping people. After graduating, I started my first job as an occupational therapist at the Rehabilitation Institute of Chicago. I found myself working mostly with patients who had suffered from a stroke, multiple sclerosis, or some other neurological disorder. I was definitely helping people, but I realized I wanted to prevent these conditions in the first place. I wanted to work with patients when they were first diagnosed in order to prevent their conditions from reaching the point at which they needed inpatient rehabilitation. I wanted to teach patients how to live healthy lives to prevent the development of certain illnesses and diseases. So I decided I would become a physician, because I figured a physician was the first one to make a diagnosis, and thus would be able to prevent decline in health. I wanted to teach people how to be healthy and prevent disease. As I was studying for the MCAT, the exam to get into medical school, I had what I call my spiritual awakening.

A friend of mine suggested that I see a Chinese doctor in Chicago's Chinatown to try to improve my circulation. Chicago winters can be brutal for someone with poor circulation. This Chinese doctor listened to my complaints, looked at my tongue, felt my pulse and prescribed some awful tasting herbs that I had to drink as a tea. He also performed acupuncture treatments to improve my blood flow. I am not sure if it was the herbs or the acupuncture, but slowly my condition improved. Around this same time, as I was getting closer to taking the MCAT, I had a long talk with two friends who were physicians. I explained that I wanted to become a doctor to spend time with my patients, listen to their stories and help people change their diets, lifestyles, and unhealthy habits. I wanted to educate people on how to take charge of their health in order to prevent disease. I told my friends about my experience with the Chinese physician and how he had improved my circulation without the use of drugs or making me move to a warmer climate. My friends related their medical school experiences, residency trainings and current practice settings. They were frustrated by insurance restrictions, the lack of time they had with patients and how their treatments nearly always boiled down to drugs and surgery. I knew at that point that conventional medical school was not for me.

So I hoped in the car with my dog in tow and headed to Austin, Texas, and Albuquerque, New Mexico, to look into acupuncture schools. After a while, I realized Chinese medicine was close, but not exactly what I was looking for when I envisioned myself working with patients. Then it happened. I was back in Chicago sipping coffee in Kopi Café on Clark Street when I opened an alternative health magazine and saw an ad for naturopathic medical school. I had never heard of naturopathic medicine, so I did some research. What I discovered was exactly what I was looking for.

This was 1996, and at that time there were only four naturopathic medical schools in the U.S. that were approved by the U.S. Department of Education: Bastyr University in Seattle, National College of Natural Medicine in Portland, Oregon, Bridgeport University in Connecticut and Southwest College of Naturopathic Medicine in Tempe, Arizona. (Currently, there is an additional naturopathic school in Lombard, Illinois, at the National University of Health Sciences, and two schools in Canada.) These are freestanding, four-year medical schools with outpatient clinical training and residency programs. The first two years are identical to conventional medical schools in terms of the basic science education, but the philosophy and foundation is unique. Naturopathic medicine focuses on using the healing powers of nature for treatments, such as botanical medicine, homeopathy, nutritional counseling, hydrotherapy, supporting the body with nutrients, and physical medicine. I didn't realize until I was in school that naturopaths are trained to adjust the spine like a chiropractor or osteopath. Naturopathic physicians also use pharmaceutical drugs and perform minor surgery when necessary, blending the best of both conventional and alternative medicine. The foundation and philosophy is rooted in treating the underlying cause and not the symptom. This was what I had been looking for, and it felt right, so off I went to Portland, Oregon, to attend naturopathic medical school.

Currently there are 15 states, plus the District of Columbia, Puerto Rico and the Virgin Islands, that license naturopathic physicians in the U.S. In these states, naturopathic doctors are required to graduate from an accredited four-year residential naturopathic medical school and pass an extensive postdoctoral board examination (NPLEX) in order to receive a license. For information about the Naturopathic Physicians Licensing Examination Board (NPLEX) and the North American Board of Naturopathic Examiners (NABNE), and for a list of naturopathic medical schools, states that license naturopathic medicine, and to find a doctor in your area, visit: *www.naturopathic.org*.

My interest in women's health was evident from the start. During my clinical training portion of medical school, I began specializing in gynecology and women's health. I couldn't help wondering why women are always going to the doctor. Why are most women's health problems related to hormones? When I began seeing patients as a medical student, some of my questions were answered. One day, a woman in her forties came to see me for what she described as allergies. Every time she walked down the detergent/cleaning aisle at her local grocery store, she experienced a headache, became fatigued, and felt short of breath and shaky. She began to experience these same symptoms whenever she smelled someone's perfume or cologne, was exposed to auto exhaust, or was in a building without fresh air. She had a condition called multiple chemical sensitivity (MCS). This is a condition known to be related to exposure to environmental toxins.[2] As I began to research her condition, I learned how synthetic chemicals and other environmental substances can mimic hormones in the body, especially estrogen. I learned that chemicals can be harmful, or toxic, to humans, and can contribute to illness and disease.

Another patient came to see me for unexplained infertility. She had already been to an OB/GYN and a reproductive endocrinologist. No one could figure out why she and her husband could not get pregnant. She had gone through two rounds of fertility treatments with drugs and intrauterine insemination to no avail. I was eventually able to link toxins she had been exposed to while living next door to a gas station to her infertility. After testing her for solvents and heavy metals, I put her through a treatment plan designed to remove toxins stored in the body. Eventually, she was able to conceive.

Next was a patient with endometriosis, which causes very painful menstrual cramps. Her OB/GYN wanted to put her on birth control pills to treat the symptoms of painful menstrual cycles, but she did not want to do this because she and her husband wanted to start having kids. I linked her endometriosis to chemicals found in plastics, cosmetics, and pesticides, known as estrogen mimickers. After taking her through a program to remove toxins from her body, her symptoms of endometriosis disappeared. Next it was a patient with fibroids, then a patient with polycystic ovarian syndrome (PCOS), and numerous patients with thyroid dysfunction. All these conditions were linked to toxins in the environment.

Over the years, I have seen hundreds of women with various health conditions linked to exposure to toxins. These are common toxins that we come in contact with every day through our food, water, air, cleaning products, cosmetics, and plastics. Sometimes we don't even know we are in contact with these harmful substances. We are flooded with chemicals in our environment and are exposed to low doses of them every day. We are exposed at home, at work, in our cars, and when we travel. We are essentially exposed to them nonstop. But so what? Aren't these exposures in such small amounts that they don't harm us? Don't they just pass through our bodies anyway? Recent research shows that low-dose, everyday exposure to toxins in our environment can indeed build up in our bodies over time and affect our health.[3] Chemicals can affect our hormonal systems, immune systems and neurological systems.[4]

Currently, in the United States, there is a 'green' movement underway. People are talking about doing things that are good for the earth and for the environment. I would like everyone to stop and ask, is better for the environment really better for you? If a piece of wood is made from recycled material but is also coated in a toxic sealant or treated with arsenic, is it really better? If a compact florescent light bulb is more energy-efficient and cost-efficient but still poses a risk for mercury exposure when it is crushed or broken, is that a good thing? The point is, the word 'green' doesn't necessarily mean it is good for your health. Your health is what this book is about.

One might ask, 'If we are all exposed to chemicals on some level every day, then why do some people become ill and others do not?' The explanation as to why toxins affect us all differently lies in our genes, or in other words, in our genetic make-up. This will be explained in depth in later chapters, but basically, some of us are genetically set up to have trouble clearing toxins from the body. Normally, our bodies are well designed to handle chemical assault on a small scale. Later I will discuss the body's natural defense mechanisms and explain how some of us hold on to toxins and others don't. Those who hold on to the toxins and don't clear them from the body tend to be the ones who develop health conditions linked to chemicals in the environment.

How do we know if these chemical exposures are affecting our health and what can we do about it? First, we need to educate ourselves about what these chemicals are, how we are exposed to them on a daily basis, and what types of symptoms and illnesses can be related to exposure. Then we can decide what to do about it.

In the following chapters, I will explain what I mean by environmental toxins and give examples of the most common ones you come in contact with every day. I will list ways in which you are exposed to these toxins so they can be avoided. Next, I will discuss various women's health conditions and cite evidence from scientific research that links toxins to each condition. I will explain what methods of testing are available to determine which toxins are stored in your body and explain my method for removing these chemicals from the body. I will outline an 8-week detoxification plan that you can do at home.

My practice focuses on women's health and environmental medicine. Whether it is breast cancer, endometriosis, fibroids, infertility, miscarriage, thyroid dysfunction, or other hormonal imbalances, I try to discover the cause and not just treat the symptom. Over the years, I have discovered a link between chemicals in our environment and women's health problems. My goal is to spread the word that there is something you can do to prevent these health problems and remove toxins from your body.

CHAPTER I
HOW TOXIC ARE YOU?

An environmental toxin sounds like something that only people who are in certain jobs might come across. Occupations such as industrial workers, agricultural workers, or workers in a hair salon would be considered at risk for chemical exposure. These types of occupational exposures are called high-dose exposures due to the amount of chemicals these workers come in contact with each day. That means that these workers are exposed to higher-than-normal amounts of chemicals while at work. In the past, scientists used to think the dose made the poison, and that only high-dose exposure to chemicals at work could cause health problems. The truth is that every person is exposed to chemicals every day by simply living an ordinary life. You are exposed by eating food, breathing the air, drinking water, driving a car, traveling on a plane, using certain products in and around your home, going to work, having a hobby, remodeling a home, moving into a new home, buying a new car, showering or taking a bath, putting on makeup, coloring your hair, and, well, pretty much just living. It is important to know how you are exposed in order to make healthy lifestyle decisions and avoid these exposures.

A toxin is any substance or chemical that creates an irritating or harmful effect in the body. Chemicals can get into the body by absorption through the skin, which can happen whenever you touch something or something touches you. They also get into your body by inhalation through the nose and mouth, and by ingestion when you eat or drink something. Most toxins are very lipophilic, meaning they are fat-loving; these are also called fat-soluble compounds, and they love to hang out in your fat. Your body cannot easily break down fat-soluble compounds, and thus they are stored and hang around for a long time. Toxins can cross the placental and blood-brain barrier, and are passed from mother to baby in-utero and during breast-feeding.[1]

The rain-barrel effect

Toxicity or toxic overload occurs when you are exposed to more than your body can break down and eliminate. Dr. William Rea makes the analogy to a rain barrel, where drops of rain slowly fill a barrel. If enough rain is collected in the barrel and it's never emptied, then the rain barrel eventually overflows, it starts to rust, bacteria grows in the water, or mold forms. This is similar to people's daily exposure to toxins. A small amount of one toxin plus a small amount of another toxin builds up in your body and eventually some illness or disease develops because the body overflows with toxins.

But what happens to all those raindrops inside the rain barrel? Does it mix together and blend into the same rainwater? Most likely, since it is all essentially rain. The same is not true for toxins mixing together in the body. Daily exposure to toxins that build up in the body can be very different types of compounds. One might be a heavy metal, such as mercury, another might be a pesticide, such as DDT, and another might be a solvent from gasoline, such as xylene. These different compounds by themselves are harmful. But what happens in the body when they all mix together?

Different compounds can interact with each other once inside the body. This is called a synergistic effect, and it has recently become an area of study. In the past, when toxins were tested at low doses to see if they caused harm to humans, they were tested one compound at a time. Recently, researchers have been testing how toxins at low doses interact with each other in the body. They have found that a chemical once thought to be safe at a low-dose is indeed not safe when combined with another chemical at a low-dose.[2] This cumulative or synergistic effect happens in our lives every day. You don't live in a world where you are exposed to only one toxin at a time. You eat, drink, and breathe all day, every day; thus, you are exposed to numerous compounds all at once. Both a rain barrel and the body need to be emptied frequently in order to stay healthy. The chapter on treatment will explain how to remove chemicals from the body.

Body burden

In theory, your body is set up to remove unwanted toxins. Once you are exposed, they enter the bloodstream and go to the liver, where they get metabolized and broken down. The broken-down byproducts are then eliminated from your body through the kidneys, stool and the skin. You remove the byproducts through urination, having a bowel movement, and perspiring. Some people can't metabolize and remove toxins very well. They are born with genetic changes in the enzymes in their liver, and they don't break down the toxins. Some people have pre-existing disease or health conditions affecting their livers, kidneys and bowels, making elimination difficult. Conditions such as fatty liver disease, cirrhosis, Crohns' disease, ulcerative colitis, diarrhea, constipation, poor perspiration, having only one kidney, and other health problems can decrease the body's ability to remove toxins. Such factors make these people more susceptible to low-dose exposures of chemicals simply because they can't break them down and get rid of them easily. Then there are people whose bodies function just fine, but they have been exposed to so many toxins or at such a high dose that they just can't clear them.

Let me remind you of the rain barrel analogy. A drop of rain, a drop of rain, and a drop of rain over time will fill up that rain barrel, and if it is not drained or emptied, then the water overflows. It is the same with your body. A little bit of this toxin plus a little bit of that toxin builds up in your body, and eventually your body overflows with a disease or illness.

You store toxins in your fat tissue (adipose), organs, bones and cells. Most toxins are fat-soluble and can remain there for years, affecting the hormonal system, immune system and neurological system.

So, how many chemicals are really in our bodies? Studies have been conducted on healthy people, sick people, newborn babies, people who work with toxins and people who live toxic-free lifestyles to see what is stored in their bodies. These studies are called body-burden studies. Levels of toxins are measured in the blood, urine, breast milk, or fat samples. (Yes, you can actually take a chunk of fat and measure what toxins are stored there.) Breast milk contains toxins and lactation is a method of excreting chemicals from the body. Mothers with high levels of toxins in their bodies will remove toxins through breast-feeding. This might sound like a good way for a woman to remove chemicals from her body, but the problem is that the toxins go into the baby receiving the breast milk. Toxins are also passed through the placental barrier. So again, mothers with toxins in their bodies will pass them to the baby in the womb.

A study by the Environmental Working Group (EWG) as part of the Human Toxome Project set out to discover how many of these chemicals actually stay in the body.[3] The study looked at the blood and urine of 55 adults. They were tested for 528 different chemicals that we are exposed to on a daily basis through ordinary living. All 55 participants had chemicals in their body, and 438 of the 528 chemicals tested for were found. Another study done by EWG looked at the umbilical cord blood of 10 newborn babies. It was tested for 413 chemicals. All 10 newborns had chemicals in their umbilical cord blood, and 287 of the 413 chemicals tested for were found.[3]

In 2010, the Centers for Disease Control (CDC) released the Fourth Report on Human Exposure to Environmental Chemicals. You can read the Fourth Report at *www.cdc.gov/ExposureReport*. It looked at 212 environmental chemicals in the blood and urine of 2,400 people in the U.S. from 2005 to 2006.[4] It included data from the previous three reports that spanned the periods of 1999 to 2000, 2001 to 2002, and 2003 to 2004. The Fourth Report found traces of commonly used chemicals in the bodies of most of the 2,400 study participants.[4]

For example:

Polybrominated diphenylethers (PBDEs) are flame-retardants that accumulate in the environment and in human fat tissue. One type of polybrominated diphenyl ether, BDE-47, was found in the serum of nearly all of the 2,400 participants.[4]

Bisphenol-A (BPA), a component in plastic bottles and the lining of metal food cans, may have potential reproductive toxicity. CDC scientists found Bisphenol-A in more than 90% of the urine samples representative of the U.S. population.[4]

Another example of widespread human exposure included perfluorooctanoic acid (PFOA), which is a byproduct of perchlorate chemicals and is used to create non-stick coatings in pots and pans. Most participants had measurable levels of it in their bodies. PFOAs are also used to manufacture fireworks, explosives, flares, and rocket propellant. Low-level exposure to perchlorate has been under investigation by many scientists in recent years. For decades, scientists have known that large medical doses of perchlorate affect thyroid function. The Fourth Report shows that all participants have detectable perchlorate in their urine.[4]

States have started to perform their own tests so they can pass legislation to restrict the use of some chemicals. In 2005, ten Washington state residents agreed to have their hair, blood, and urine tested for the presence of toxic chemicals as part of an investigative study by the Toxic-Free Legacy Coalition. They were tested for phthalates (a chemical in plastics), Polybrominated diphenylethers, lead, arsenic, mercury, pesticides and perfluorinated chemicals. Every person tested had at least 26 chemicals and some had as many as 39 of the toxic chemicals. These toxins came from everyday exposure through regular activities and use of products.[5] California is leading the way with body-burden studies and regulation of environmental toxins. A group called the California Body Burden Campaign investigates the amount of chemicals stored in the body of the average person.[6]

You can watch the news or surf the Internet and find numerous body burden studies that have taken place in the United States. Even famous people are getting tested as part of a research project or news report. There is one about Bill Moyers, a well known journalist. As part of a study on chemicals in the human body sponsored by the Mount Sinai School of Medicine in New York, samples of Bill Moyers' blood and urine were analyzed. Much to his surprise, eighty-four distinct toxic chemicals were found in his body.[7]

The October 2006 issue of National Geographic ran a story called "Pollution Within" that discusses the number of chemicals the average person is exposed to each day and how these chemicals build up in the body. National Geographic paid for journalist David Ewing Duncan to undergo testing to determine his body burden of 320 chemicals. The tests consisted of blood and urine samples and cost around $15,000. The results are staggering; of the 320 chemicals tested for, 165 were found in the journalist. *http://ngm. nationalgeographic.com/2006/10/toxic-people/duncan-text*

Reporter David Ewing Duncan's results from National Geographic, Oct 2006:

	Tested	Found
PCBs	209	97
PBDEs	40	25
Pesticides	28	16
Dioxins	17	10
Phthalates	7	7
PFAs	13	7
Metals	4	3
BPA	2	0

These are a few examples of how people in the U.S. are exposed to toxins that build up in the body. These are people living ordinary lives, not people at high risk for exposure to chemicals based on a particular job, hobby or living situation. If you were to be tested, it is estimated you would have over 200 chemicals stored in your body. But how much is too much? At what amount is a chemical stored in the body a cause for concern? The Centers for Disease Control has set safe limits for the amount of chemicals we are exposed to. I refer to these limits when working with patients.

Remember, just because a chemical is present in the body doesn't necessarily mean it has caused disease and illness. Under the "Conditions" section of this book, I outline what chemicals have been scientifically proven to be linked to women's health conditions. It is important to know how you are exposed in order to make healthy lifestyle decisions and avoid these exposures. The chemicals stored in the body will affect your health in time. Some of the exposure happens before you are even born and can't be avoided. However, most of the exposure happens during your lifetime. Educating yourself on how you are exposed, and learning how to remove these chemicals with an 8-week detoxification plan, are important steps in improving your health.

CHAPTER II
HOW ARE YOU EXPOSED?

Food

Let's start with food. We have all heard the phase 'you are what you eat.' But when you consider the amount of toxins that you ingest primarily through eating, the phrase is frightening. You ingest pesticides by eating fruit, vegetables and dairy products. There are pesticides in your wine and olive oil. You are exposed to mercury, polychlorinated biphenyls (PCBs), and dioxins by eating fish. You are exposed to phthalates and bisphenol-A through food stored in plastic, cooked in plastic, handled with plastic gloves, and covered with plastic cling wrap. There is cadmium, arsenic and lead in some foods. You are exposed to heterocyclic amines and polycyclic aromatic hydrocarbons while cooking foods at high temperatures or on the grill. It may seem overwhelming, but if you know what you are being exposed to when you eat, you can learn how to avoid exposure by merely changing your eating habits.

The general rule of thumb is that eating organic fruits and vegetables, fish low in mercury, minimal amounts of animal products (which must be organic), eliminating plastics from food, and changing how we prepare food will significantly reduce the amount of toxins ingested or inhaled.

Pesticides

The average person in America is exposed to pesticides through food. Fruits and vegetables sitting in the produce department waiting to be eaten have been tested for pesticide residue, and the results show high amounts.[1] Pesticides on foods are mainly organophosphate pesticides. Throughout this book, the term "pesticides" will include insecticides and herbicides whether they are organophosphates, organochlorine, carbamate or pyrethroids. This is done to keep it simple. See the glossary for a more detailed definition of toxins.

The Environmental Working Group (EWG) is a nonprofit organization consisting of scientists, engineers, policymakers, lawyers and others committed to providing the public with information on the environment and health. They have conducted studies showing pesticide residue on non-organic produce in the supermarket. Here is a summary of their research.[1]

Findings from the Environmental Working Group

The non-organic fruits and vegetables with the highest levels of pesticides are:

- Peaches
- Strawberries
- Apples
- Domestic blueberries
- Nectarines
- Cherries
- Imported grapes
- Celery
- Sweet bell peppers
- Spinach
- Kale
- Collard greens
- Potatoes

The non-organic fruits and vegetables with the lowest levels of pesticides are:

◆ Onions
◆ Sweet corn
◆ Sweet peas
◆ Asparagus
◆ Cabbage
◆ Eggplant
◆ Sweet potatoes
◆ Avocados
◆ Pineapple
◆ Mangoes
◆ Kiwi
◆ Domestic cantaloupe
◆ Watermelon
◆ Grapefruit
◆ Honeydew

Pesticides are present as residue in more than just fruits and vegetables. They are in peanut butter, beef, butter, bread, ice cream, olive oil, and eggs.[2,3] This is due to the widespread agricultural use of pesticides, which is a broad term for herbicides, insecticides and fungicides. Such chemicals are also used in and around homes. Pesticides can persist for years in the soil, contaminate groundwater and drinking water, and can accumulate up the food chain. Pesticides can end up in places they were never intended to be due to wind drift, meaning the wind carries them to nearby fields, homes, and schools. Studies show pesticides are present in non-organic meat, dairy and eggs due to these effects.[4]

Fish

It is generally agreed upon that eating fish has positive health benefits because they are full of omega-3 fatty acids. Fish that is wild, or caught in the wild, means it is from the ocean, rivers, lakes or steams. The downside to wild fish is that it is full of mercury. Mercury comes in various forms in the environment. There is organic, elemental, and inorganic mercury. Organic mercury includes methyl, ethyl, alkyl, and phenyl mercury. Methylmercury is the form found in wild and farmed fish.

So how does mercury get into our food? Mercury is released into the air from coal-burning power plants, the incineration of medical and municipal waste, and other industrial sources. It travels as air pollution and drops back into the atmosphere over rivers, lakes, streams and the ocean, where fish are exposed to it and convert it into methylmercury. The mercury accumulates up the food chain until it reaches you. The more fish you eat, the higher levels of methylmercury in your body. Mercury is known to affect the nervous system and a woman's reproductive system and the developing fetus.[5]

On October 29, 2007, USA Today Online published an interactive map of where in the U.S. mercury was being released into the air, and where in the U.S. fish had the highest levels of mercury.[6] The East and West Coast states and the Great Lake states were the states that emitted the most mercury into the air. It is no coincidence that these states had the most contaminated fish. Visit the USA Today website to get a better understanding of which fish are not safe to eat in your state. *http://www.usatoday.com/news/health/2007-10-29-mercury-cover_N.htm*

Here are some examples of fish high in mercury, based on location in the United States:

California

- Bass (all types)
- Bat ray
- Black crappie
- Brown bullhead
- California halibut
- Carp
- Catfish
- Chinook salmon
- Clams
- Crayfish
- Gold fish
- Jacksmelt
- Minnow
- Shark (all types)
- Rainbow trout
- Red rock crab
- Shellfish
- Shiner perch
- Sturgeon
- Trout
- Sunfish (all types)

Illinois

- Bass (all types)
- Crappie
- Carp and crappie
- Flathead catfish
- Muskellunge
- Northern Pike
- Souger
- Walleye

In general it is advised to avoid all large, fatty fish that are high on the food chain. Do not eat swordfish, shark, king mackerel or tilefish and limit albacore tuna to one meal (6 ounces) a month.

Fish lowest in mercury:

+ Blue crab (mid-Atlantic)
+ Croaker
+ Fish sticks
+ Flounder (summer)
+ Haddock
+ Trout (farmed)
+ Salmon (wild Pacific)
+ Shrimp - but high in inorganic arsenic

Remember, it is not the fish's fault it is full of mercury. The mercury comes from man-made industries that pollute the air and water and eventually our food. Electing officials who are willing to impose tighter regulations and writing your local members of Congress and Senate and other state officials is a step in the right direction. Action needs to be taken!

So if wild fish is contaminated with mercury, why don't we just eat farmed fish? Farmed fish has its own problems. Most fish sold in supermarkets and served at restaurants is farmed, unless it specifically advertises that it is wild. Farmed fish are essentially raised in captivity and fed fishmeal and fish oil manufactured from small, open-sea fish. There are numerous studies documenting that farmed fish are contaminated with pesticides, dioxins and PCBs.[7, 8]

Plastic and food

Plastic contains compounds such as phthalates and bisphenol-A (BPA), which are designed to make it durable, flexible, and hard. When food is stored in plastic or wrapped in plastic wrap, it also contains these compounds because they can leach out of plastic into food. BPA is used in the manufacture of polycarbonate plastic and is in the lining of metal food cans. Many plastic water bottles are made of BPA. It is a known environmental estrogen and has adverse health effects in both men and women. These effects are described in the chapter on health conditions, and each chemical is explained in detail in the glossary.

BPA can leach out of plastic water bottles and metal food cans and build up in our bodies over time. Heating of cans that are lined with BPA can cause increased leaching. The presence of acidic or basic foods or beverages can also increase leaching. The repeated washing of polycarbonate plastics also causes BPA to leach into food and drink.[9] A 2008 study published in *The Journal of the American Medical Association* links BPA to an increased risk of heart disease, diabetes and liver problems.[10] California and Connecticut recently enacted a law removing BPA from children's toys.

Another chemical found in plastic is phthalates. Many of the foods we eat come stored in plastic or wrapped in plastic wrap, from the soft plastic tubs that hold butter, to plastic milk cartons, the condiments and dressings containers, and the plastic wrap that preserves cheese. All of these could be leaching phthalates into your food. Plastic beverage bottles can leach phthalates into your water, juice and soda. Studies have found phthalates in milk, butter, margarine, vegetable oils, and cheeses.[11] Buying milk, condiments, dressing and other foods in glass containers instead of plastic helps avoid exposure to these compounds.

Phthalates can even get into our food if handled by a food preparer wearing plastic gloves.[12] But what we hear about in the media most often is plastic water bottles. One form of phthalates is in plastic beverage bottles. Phthalates can leach out of the bottle, causing our beverages to be another possible source of exposure to toxins.[13]

Plastics are a common source of daily low-dose exposure to environmental toxins that, for the most part, can be avoided by the choices you make at the store. In the chapter discussing specific diseases, it will become clear how these compounds are harmful to your health.

Heavy metals in our food

How do heavy metals, such as arsenic, cadmium, lead and mercury, get into our food? We have already discussed mercury in the section about wild fish, but what about the other metals, and is mercury present in foods other than fish? Heavy metals can be found in grains, flour, pasta, and vegetables due to contaminated soil and fertilizer. In the United States, sewage sludge is commonly used as fertilizer and may be contaminated with heavy metals. Accumulation of heavy metals in the soil due to repeated application of sewage sludge as a plant nutrient source is common. In some cases increased amounts of heavy metals in plants are found as a consequence. For example; the sludge's content of arsenic seems to be easily available to plants. Fungicides containing mercury and runoff from industry-polluted waters are other sources of heavy metal contamination. The amount of heavy metals in your vegetables depends on the soil conditions and fertilizer. Cadmium is the most common contaminant. The U.S. does not place a limit on the amount of cadmium and lead that can be present in fertilizer.[14, 15]

Food preparation: Manning the grill

Cooking meats at high temperatures can create chemicals that are not ordinarily present in meats. When you eat the meat, you ingest these chemicals, which are known carcinogens. It is not just beef that creates these chemicals; it is all muscle meats, including fish, chicken, turkey, pork and beef. These chemicals are called heterocyclic amines (HCAs), and are linked to cancer, according to the National Cancer Institute. When muscle meats are cooked at high temperatures, 17 different HCAs can be produced. The higher the temperature the meat is cooked at, the higher the number of HCAs that are produced. Frying, broiling and barbecuing produce the greatest quantity of this chemical, since these methods of cooking techniques are all performed at very high temperatures.

Another chemical released during the grilling of muscle meats is polycyclic aromatic hydrocarbon (PAH). It can be produced in someone's backyard or in a manufacturing facility where smoked meats are produced. These chemicals are also dangers to your health and will be linked to specific health conditions in later chapters. The theme for cooking meats (which need to be organic, of course) is 'low and slow.' Cook meats at a low temperature over a longer period of time, just like when you use a crock pot.

At this point, you may feel like there is nothing safe to eat. That is simply not true, and in both the chapter on avoidance and the chapter on how to remove toxins from your body, I will outline ways to eat healthfully, avoid chemicals in food and use foods to remove toxins from the body.

Water

Water is another source of exposure of environmental toxins. Water that comes into your home is used for more than drinking, and toxins can enter the body through ingestion by mouth, absorption through the skin, and inhalation. Toxins are in the water you use to take a shower or a bath, to brush your teeth, to wash your clothes and dishes, and to cook. Some people think that drinking bottled water is a safer alternative, but is it?

Concern over the drinking water in this country is nothing new. In the 1970s, the Environmental Protection Agency and Congress passed two pieces of legislation to protect your waterways and drinking water. The Clean Water Act of 1972 maintains the physical, chemical and biological integrity of this nation's waterways, and the Safe Drinking Water Act of 1974 controls drinking water contamination through multiple regulations.

The source of drinking water varies greatly depending on where you live. Freshwater sources include rivers, lakes, and streams, which accumulate through rainfall and snowmelt. This accounts for what is known as surface water. Groundwater is another source of drinking water; it accumulates through rainfall that seeps into the soil until it reaches a layer of rock. This water, once it saturates the soil and collects in the rock, can flow into a river or lake or an aquifer. Some cities have underground aquifers that hold groundwater in a spring or well.[1]

No matter where your drinking water comes from—surface water or groundwater—there is a chance it can be contaminated. This is why the EPA created regulations and standards for making sure drinking water is free of toxins. The EPA regulates public water, not water from a private source. Typically, an independent company manages private sources of drinking water and is responsible for treating it and removing harmful chemicals.

What types of contaminants are in our drinking water? There can be bacteria and viruses, which are typically removed through a city's disinfection and filtration processes. There can be agricultural and industrial runoff, leading to high levels of pesticides and heavy metals in the water. Volatile organic compounds (VOCs), chlorine disinfection byproducts, and medications can all be found in the water supply as well. I will highlight a few recent findings regarding our nation's drinking water that made headline news.

In March 2008, the Associated Press released the results of an investigation into pharmaceutical drugs in our tap water. In Philadelphia, the researchers found 56 drugs in the tap water, including pain medication, antibiotics, and medication for cholesterol, asthma, epilepsy and heart problems. In Southern California, 18.5 million people's water had anti-epileptic and anti-anxiety medications, and a sex hormone was found in San Francisco's water. Washington, D.C.'s water was found to have six different drugs. All of the water tested had already gone through the city's treatment facility.

In May of 2008, the city of Phoenix, Arizona, found high levels of Trihalomethanes (THMs) in the drinking water. THMs are a byproduct of the disinfection process. Most cities use chlorine to disinfect the water. The THMs include chloroform, bromoform, bromodichloromethane, and dibromochloromethane. You are exposed to these through drinking water, showering and bathing. The THMs are associated with adverse birth outcomes, and they are known to cause cancer.[2]

Agriculture and industry are two means by which volatile organic compounds, heavy metals and pesticides end up in your drinking water. For many years, industry dumped chemicals into lakes, rivers and streams, polluting surface water. Both agricultural run-off and industrial contamination have also affected groundwater. Recently, in Scottsdale, Arizona, and Paradise Valley, Arizona, the Motorola Company contaminated groundwater with trichloroethylene (TCE). It happened in October 2007 and again in January 2008. Motorola leaked TCE into the drinking water that serves Scottsdale and Paradise Valley. The cities instructed people to drink bottled water until the problem was corrected. I was shocked that residents were not advised against bathing and showering in the contaminated water. Motorola ended up having to pay a very large fine for dumping the cancer-causing toxin into the city's water supply.

These are just a few examples of recent news reports of environmental toxins turning up in the water. Many of the toxins are cancer-causing and are related to birth defects and other health concerns. Get your water tested by an independent company to find out what is in your water. In the avoidance section of this book, I will address water filtration in the home so you can learn how to properly clean the water you and your family drink and use to bathe or shower. There are easy and inexpensive ways to remove chemicals from your water at home and at work.

Plastic water bottles

When I discuss water as a source of environmental toxins, people tell me they don't have to worry because they drink filtered water out of plastic bottles. But there is evidence to show that the plastic leaches harmful chemicals into the water, thus exposing the drinker to environmental toxins.

When I talk about plastic water bottles, I am referring to all plastic beverage bottles. It doesn't matter if it is water or soda or juice that is inside. Plastic bottles are made with chemicals known as plasticizers. Their purpose is to make plastic strong and flexible. There are two main forms of plastic that make up plastic water bottles: polyvinyl chloride plastics (PVC) and polycarbonate plastics. PVC contains the most commonly used commercial plasticizer known as phthalates. Polycarbonate plastics contain a chemical called bisphenol-A (BPA).

Both phthalates and bisphenol-A are known hormone disrupting chemicals, often called "hormone mimicking compounds." Studies show that both phthalates and BPA have adverse health effects in humans and are linked to infertility, premature puberty, asthma, allergies, menstrual cycle irregularities, breast cancer and prostate cancer.[3,4,5]

But what is in the average plastic beverage bottle? Some bottles are soft and flexible and crunch when they're empty and you squeeze them. Some are firm, sturdy, and strong. Are they all the same? Do they all have these harmful chemicals? The answer is complicated, but the number on the bottom of the bottle can be used as a general guide as to what chemical plasticizer is in the bottle.

Flip that bottle over

#1 PETE or PET (polyethylene terephthalate): Used for most water and soda bottles. The ingredients include resins made from methane, xylene and ethylene combined with the chemical ethylene glycol and other chemicals. These have flame retardants and UV stabilizers added.

#2 HDPE (high density polyethylene): Used for cloudy milk and water jugs and opaque food bottles. Its resins are made from ethylene and propylene resins and have flame retardants added. When burned, HDPE bottles release formaldehyde and dioxin if chlorine was used during manufacturing.

#3 PVC or V (Polyvinyl chloride): Used in some cling wrap, plastic wrap around foods such as cheese, soft beverage bottles, plastic containers, plumbing pipes, children's toys, vinyl windows, shower curtains, shades, blinds and many other items. They create toxic byproducts when burned, such as PCB's and dioxins. They are made from petroleum resins and have flame retardants added.

#4 LDPE (low density polyethylene): Used in plastic grocery bags, plastic wrap, bubble wrap, dry-cleaning bags, and flexible lids. Its resins are made from ethylene and propylene resins and have flame retardants added. When burned, HDPE bottles release formaldehyde and dioxin if chlorine was used during manufacturing.

#5 PP (polypropylene): Used in yogurt cups, some baby bottles, screw-on caps, toys, and drinking straws. Its resins are made from ethylene and propylene resins and have flame retardants added. When burned, HDPE bottles release formaldehyde and dioxin if chlorine was used during manufacturing.

#6 PS (polystyrene): Used in egg cartons, foam meat trays, clear takeout containers, plastic cutlery, toys, cups, and CD containers. Its resins are made from ethylene and propylene resins and have flame retardants added. When burned, they release styrene and polyaromatic hydrocarbons.

#7 Other (usually polycarbonate): Used in five-gallon water bottles, some baby bottles, and the lining of metal food cans. They create toxic byproducts when burned, such as PCBs and dioxins. They are made from petroleum resins and have flame retardants added.

In general, polystyrene plastic leaches the solvent styrene, polycarbonate plastic leaches bisphenol-A, and polyvinyl chloride and polyethylene terephthalate leach phthalates. This accounts for #1, #3, #6, and #7 above. The nonprofit Berkeley Ecology Center found that the manufacture of PETE uses large amounts of energy and resources and generates toxic emissions and pollutants. The remaining plastics—#2, #4, and #5 above—may leach chemicals too, but there are no studies to show that they leach chemicals known to cause hormone disruption in humans. They would be the safest option.[6]

Currently, manufacturers are phasing out BPA from the hard-plastic water bottles. I was recently in an outdoor store called REI and noticed all the hard water bottles said BPA free. This is a huge step in the right direction. Other steps would be to drink water filtered at home out of a glass or metal container. These containers can be found at outdoor and health foods stores.

Air

Have you ever gone on vacation to the ocean or up in the mountains or to a scarcely populated area and noticed that the air seemed clean, crisp and refreshing? You likely noticed that when you returned home to your city, the air just wasn't as pure. Well, you were not imagining it. The air you breathe is loaded with environmental toxins and is contributing to health problems. You can go days, even weeks, without food and hours without water, but without air, you would be dead in minutes. Polluted air won't kill you immediately, but it could over time. It is the job of the Environmental Protection Agency to make sure that doesn't happen.

In 1970, Congress created the Environmental Protection Agency (EPA), and a law was passed called the Clean Air Act in an effort to improve the air quality in the U.S. It was created to protect against common pollutants, including ground level ozone (smog), carbon monoxide, sulfur dioxide, nitrogen dioxide, lead, and particulate soot. State governments had to develop plans to meet the heath standards by a specific date. The Clean Air Act was amended in 1977 and again in 1990 to make even tougher standards in favor of clean air. Air pollution not only affects humans, but it also damages animals, plants, rivers, lakes, oceans, trees, and crops. It damages statues, cars, buildings, homes, the ozone layer and eventually the earth. Air pollution can cause or irritate asthma, allergies, and other respiratory problems. It also can cause cancer, reproductive problems, skin irritation, and as you will learn later, a host of other illnesses.[1]

The Clean Air Act sets limits on toxins in the air created by chemical plants, utilities, agriculture spraying, automobiles, buses, airplanes, forest fires, solid waste disposal, active volcanoes, and others polluters. There are numerous toxins that pollute the environment. Six common ones are particulate matter, ozone, carbon monoxide, sulfur oxides, nitrogen oxides, and lead. I will discuss the main two pollutants, particulate matter and ozone.[2]

Particulate matter (PM) is very fine dust, soot, and smoke that is formed when fuels such as coal, wood, or oil are burned. For example, gases from motor vehicles, electric power generation, and industrial facilities react with sunlight and water vapor to form particles. Particles may also come from fireplaces, wood stoves, unpaved roads, and construction sites, and may be blown into the air by the wind. PM causes irritation in the lungs, smog or that haze in the air, reducing visibility, and dirtying buildings and structures.[2,3]

Smog not only reduces visibility, making it difficult to see the natural beauty surrounding our cities, it also causes health problems. The main component of smog is ground-level ozone, which is something we create. Ozone is formed by cars burning gasoline, jet fuel, petroleum refineries, chemical manufacturing plants, and other industrial facilities. It is also formed by volatile organic compounds (VOCs), which are in our paints, cleaning products and more.[2,3]

Other chemicals in our outdoor air are carbon monoxide from car and truck exhaust, sulfur dioxide from cars and industrial emissions, polyaromatic hydrocarbons from cigarette smoke, fireplaces, grilling meat outdoors, and again, auto exhaust. There are also other pollutants in our air, such as heavy metals and solvents from refineries and other industrial plants. Farming and agriculture creates nitrous oxide from nitrogen fertilizers, which can contribute to the generation of ozone in our environment.[3]

As you can see, most outdoor air pollution is man-made. The recent emphasis on global warming is not only important for our future climate, but also because by placing limits on factors that contribute to global warming, we will improve air quality and thus improve our health. These air pollutants can cause allergies, asthma, immune and reproductive problems, and problems with our heart and lungs.[3] Many cities have poor air quality. You can have a say in the air quality of the city you live in by simply writing your local city, county and state representatives and demanding that they place limits on emissions and implement other known methods of improving outdoor air.

I better stay indoors

Recently, during an office visit with a patient, I was describing outdoor air pollution and how it could be affecting her health. After I described the possible toxins she was exposed to each day just from breathing, she said, "Well, I better just stay indoors." Unfortunately, indoor air is more toxic than outdoor air. Since most people spend 90% of their time indoors, either at home or at work, it is frightening to think that indoor air might be making us sick. But what actually causes indoor air pollution? Again, most of it is created by bringing items that contains toxins into the home. The chemicals are slowly released into the home; this is called off-gassing. For example, you might pick up your clothes from the drycleaner and bring them home and hang them in the closet, not realizing they are releasing a common solvent used in dry-cleaning called trichloroethylene (TCE). You might buy a new mattress, which can off-gas a flame retardant that was used in making the mattress. Carpet and furniture can release formaldehyde, and you might be using a detergent or cleaning product with harmful solvents and spraying it inside your home.

Dr. Sherry Rogers describes some common sources of indoor air pollution in her book *The EI Syndrome.*

Here are a few examples:

♦   Carpet: emits formaldehyde and volatile organic compounds (VOCs)

♦   Cigarette smoke: contains numerous toxins, including solvents, heavy metals and polyaromatic hydrocarbons (PAHs)

♦   Furniture and cabinetry made of pressed wood: emits formaldehyde

♦   Paints and building materials: emits VOCs

♦   Insecticide use on pets or plants

♦   Household cleaners: VOCs

♦   Hobbies such as painting, stained glass, film developing: various toxins

♦   Auto exhaust from an attached garage: emits VOCs, PAHs

♦   Room air fresheners and candles: VOCs and solvents

♦   Unvented gas stove and gas fireplace: emits PAHs

This list is just the beginning, but you get the idea. One source of exposure to toxins that people don't often consider is their shoes. Your shoes walk across grass, cement, carpet, and flooring at the office, stores, and other places all day. Then you come home and trek those toxins and bacteria from the bottom of your shoes into your home, compromising the air quality in your home. The take home message is this: take off your shoes when you enter the house.[4]

Indoor air quality is easier to control than outdoor air, and in the chapter on avoidance, I will offer alternatives to toxic cleaning products, paints, air fresheners and other household products contributing to poor indoor air.

Products and Cosmetics

Personal hygiene products are part of your everyday life, but what we put on our body is absorbed through the skin and circulated in the blood, and this can lead to adverse health effects. Every day, we apply shampoo, body lotion, hairspray, mascara, blush, foundation, perfume, and more. Most personal care products are applied to the skin or hair and are absorbed into our body. Some are sprayed into the air and some are washed down the drain as you shower. So, how safe are these products we apply to our skin? What happens to them as they go down the drain? Do they contribute to air pollution? Detergents, cleaners, and other household products that are not for grooming are also a source of exposure to toxins. We already learned that these products contribute to indoor air pollution, but many of them contain toxins. These products have preservatives, fragrances, solvents, penetrating agents, contaminants, foaming agents and a whole host of chemicals. So how to do you know what is safe?

There is an organization called Cosmetics Info (www.cosmeticsinfo. org) that lists factual scientific information on ingredients used in cosmetics and personal care products. I spent hours on this site searching through bath products, eye makeup products, fragrance products, hair dye and coloring products, and more. It lists common ingredients in each product and then goes on to explain that each ingredient is FDA approved and safe. The site is sponsored by The Personal Care Products Council and 'member companies,' which are not listed. This means the sponsors have a financial interest in making sure consumers, mostly women, continue to buy personal care products. The site states that its purpose is to provide consumers with information needed to make informed choices about personal care products. But is the information accurate? Let's look at hair dye/color that www.cosmeticsinfo.org says is safe.

Hair dye/color

Cosmetics Info lists the common ingredients used in most salon and over-the-counter hair dye. Each ingredient is explained and deemed safe based on scientific studies and FDA approval. The entire site operates in this fashion. A personal care product is listed, the ingredients are listed and all are deemed safe or unsafe based on scientific studies, and they point out that the ingredients are FDA-approved. Now, let's look at some studies on hair color. A population-based study done in Connecticut looked at whether lifetime hair coloring products increased cancer risk. It found that women who reported using hair color products before 1980 had increased risk of non-Hodgkin's lymphoma. It was hypothesized that recent users of hair color hadn't yet developed cancer because they are still in their cancer induction or latent period.[1] It takes years for cancer to develop, and this study ended in 2002.

Research results are conflicting when it comes to covering up that grey hair, and it gets confusing for the public. Perhaps it is the type of hair dye, or it could be the length of exposure, meaning how many times a year and over how many years coloring is done. Perhaps it is genetic makeup that makes some women more susceptible than others. One group of researchers tried to answer some of these questions by doing a review of studies linking hair dye to cancer. One interesting finding was that women who use black hair dye over a prolonged period of time had increased risk for multiple myeloma and non-Hodgkin's lymphoma.[2] Now, if a woman merely went to cosmeticsinfo.org, she would believe that all hair color/dye is safe when indeed it is not. In the chapter on avoidance, I provide resources on safe alternatives to cosmetics and hair dye.

Other personal care products

So how do you know what is safe? Just because it is FDA-approved? Maybe not. Just because the Personal Care Products Council and its 'members' state it is safe? Maybe not. Recently, the nonprofit organization The Environmental Working Group (EWG) released a report called Skin Deep: A safety assessment of ingredients in personal care products. This group reviewed the ingredients in 7,500 personal care products and compared the ingredients against government lists of cancer-causing chemicals. EWG found that one in every 100 products on the market has in it a known cancer-causing ingredient. The report can be found at www.ewg.org. You can search for your favorite products by brand name, or by category, such as "eye cream".

Some toxic ingredients to be on the lookout for are:

♦ **Coal Tar:** Used in shampoos

♦ **Benzyl violet 4B:** Used in shampoo, moisturizing body bars, nail treatments and more

♦ **Formaldehyde:** Used in lotion and nail treatment

♦ **Lead acetate:** Used in hair dye

♦ **Nitrofurazone:** Used in sunless tanner

♦ **Parabens:** Used as an antimicrobial in most products

♦ **Heavy metals (lead, mercury, cadmium):** Possibly present as a contaminant

Some critics state that these chemicals are present in such low levels that they really don't get absorbed into your body, nor do they affect your health. But researchers are beginning to look into this and have discovered otherwise. At Massachusetts General Hospital Andrology Lab, 406 men undergoing a study looking at semen quality were found to have high levels of the hormone disrupting chemical phthalate in their urine. The levels of phthalates were correlated with use of cologne or aftershave 48 hours prior to urine collection. Did you know phthalates are present in cologne and aftershave?[3] Again, even at low doses, these chemicals can build up in the body and affect health.

Smells so good

What about products that have fragrance in them? Products such as perfumes, soap, detergents, lotions, creams, and fabric softeners often use a chemical compound known as nitromusk, which contains solvents. They have been found in human fat tissue and mothers' milk, but more importantly, have been found to disrupt women's hormones. These fragrances have been linked to premenstrual syndrome, anovulation and fertility problems.[4] Later in this book, I will offer healthy alternatives for cosmetics, hair dye, and more.

Hobbies

Many people have a hobby that they enjoy. A hobby may promote relaxation, may be something to do in retirement, or may simply be a way to develop a new skill. Regardless of the reason you choose to pursue a hobby, first think about what toxins are involved. Let's take refinishing furniture as an example. This hobby includes stripping, staining and then finishing an older piece of furniture to make it look new again. Chemicals are used in all parts of this process, and these chemicals release volatile organic compounds (VOCs) that you can inhale or absorb through the skin.

Here are a few other toxic hobbies, and the chemicals involved:

♦ Glazing pottery (lead, solvents)
♦ Jewelry making (cadmium, platinum)
♦ Stained glass (lead)
♦ Ceramics (lead)
♦ Film developing (chemicals with VOCs)
♦ Painting with oil-based paints (lead, VOCs)
♦ Golf (pesticides)
♦ Crafts with adhesive rubber cement and glues (solvents)
♦ Drawing using imported crayons (lead)
♦ Restoring or fixing a car (solvents and heavy metals)

Other common sources of chemical exposure you may not be aware of:

♦ Silicone breast implants (platinum)
♦ Dental sealants for composite fillings (bisphenol-A)
♦ Silver fillings, or amalgams (mercury)
♦ Air fresheners (solvents)
♦ TVs, computers, electronics (PBDE, a flame retardant)

Food and air and water, oh my!

After reading this chapter, the numerous ways we are exposed to chemicals might seem overwhelming. This chapter is simply meant to make you aware that on a daily basis, you are exposed to small amounts of chemicals from many different sources. These chemicals do build up in your body and can, over time, cause health problems. It is important to know how you are exposed to toxins so you can learn how to make healthy choices and avoid exposure. You'll find that later in the book, I dedicate an entire chapter on how to avoid exposure to chemicals. I list healthy alternatives to most personal care and cleaning products. Also, I offer options on how to filter your air and water at home. Later, I will explain how to test for the presence of chemicals in your body and how to remove them in order to prevent or reverse disease. Knowledge is power, and knowing how you are exposed will make it easier to avoid these chemicals in your daily life. Now let's look at the scientific evidence linking exposure to chemicals and common health conditions in women.

CHAPTER III
HOW DO TOXINS AFFECT WOMEN'S HEALTH?

The science is solid. Low-dose exposure to chemicals in the environment is linked to women's health conditions. While the politics appear to be stronger than the science, women are stronger than both. As more and more women become aware of the links and make healthy choices regarding food and products they buy, corporations will take note. Real change will come as women urge elected officials at all levels to take action in protecting the environment and our health. In this section, I will outline women's health conditions and the chemicals linked to them, according to scientific evidence.

Breast Cancer

When discussing which health conditions are linked to environmental factors, it is appropriate to start with breast cancer. At some point in their lives, most women worry about getting breast cancer. Every day in the news there is a story about someone famous or not-so-famous being diagnosed with breast cancer. There are foundations and organizations promoting awareness and raising money for the disease through walks, runs, and other events. Thousands of research dollars are spent trying to find a cure, improve treatments and promote early detection.

Cancer is a multi-factorial process. Genetic, immune, and environmental factors play a role. Part of what leads to cancer is damage to genes that regulate normal cell growth. This damage can be caused in part by exposure to chemicals in the environment and in part by other factors. There are known risk factors for breast cancer that are generally agreed upon throughout the medical and scientific community. They include early menarche (age of first menstrual cycle), late menopause (when the menstrual cycle stops), having a first child later in life or not having children at all, a history of a first-degree relative with breast cancer, past exposure to ionizing radiation, obesity, excess alcohol, and use of a combination of estrogen and progestin for four years or more in postmenopausal women.[1] But these factors only account for 10% to 40% of breast cancer cases. What accounts for the rest?

We may never know the full range of causes, but environmental factors must be considered. The International Agency for Research on Cancer has identified 415 known or suspected carcinogens (cancer causers) which can be viewed at *http://monographs.iarc.fr/.* Preventing exposure to individual known carcinogens may in turn prevent cancer. You can learn which environmental exposures are linked to breast cancer in order to help prevent the disease and prevent recurrence. We may not be able to pinpoint the cause of breast cancer, but we can act on what we do know and avoid exposure to carcinogens that contribute to breast cancer.

Another reason to look at breast cancer first is that we know through research that chemicals in the environment can act like estrogen in the body. Breast tissue is extremely sensitive to estrogen stimulation, which causes breast cell division. Hormones such as estrogen, progesterone, prolactin and growth hormone affect growth and functioning of the breast. More than half of breast tumors depend on estrogen. Environmental chemicals can mimic hormones and other growth factors. They also can affect how fast the body breaks down these hormones. The chemicals can affect the balance that controls breast cell division and growth.[2]

One thing to consider when addressing environmental causes of breast cancer is that although everyone is exposed to chemicals on some level every day, not everyone gets breast cancer. Certain factors play a role in whether or not environmental exposures cause breast cancer.

Such factors include:

- Timing of exposure
- The dose of the exposure
- Synergistic effect
- Duration of exposure
- Genetic polymorphisms

In the past, researchers and clinicians thought the dose or duration of the exposure was what determined whether the toxin was carcinogenic. This was driven by cases of chemical poisoning from high-dose exposure and by occupational studies where a worker was exposed for a long period of time to a toxin. New research has focused on low-dose exposure, such as through food, and the synergistic effect of being exposed to more than one chemical at a time.[3] Also, the timing of the exposure in a patient's life has proven to be critical. For example, there are higher rates of childhood and adult cancers among those exposed to chemicals in-utero.[4] Different periods of human development are more susceptible to chemical exposure than others. During pregnancy and puberty, chemicals pass through the placental barrier. A recent study showed that exposure to a pesticide called DDT early in life, during puberty, increased risk of getting breast cancer as an adult. This again outlines the importance of the critical timing of exposure.[5]

Genetic polymorphisms need to be considered when discussing why some people exposed to chemicals develop health problems and others don't. Genetic polymorphism is a difference in the DNA sequence among individuals, groups, or populations. Single

Nucleotide Polymorphisms (SNPs) are a single-base change in DNA. SNPs in enzymes that metabolize environmental toxins play an important role and may contribute to whether or not someone has health consequences from exposure to chemicals. Toxins are broken down in the liver during phase-one detoxification involving the cytochrome P450 enzymes. In phase-two of liver metabolism, toxins are further broken down through conjugation reactions. Determining patients' SNPs, along with exposure history, can help determine breast cancer risk or perhaps explain its cause in some patients. Almost every cancer has been linked to at least one genetic polymorphism and testing for SNPs should be considered in all patients with breast cancer. (More about this in the chapter on testing.)

Breast Cancer and SNPs

According to an article in the April 2005 issue of the *International Journal of Cancer*, women with an N-acetyltransferase 2 (NAT2) polymorphism have an increased risk of breast cancer. N-acetyltransferase 2 is an enzyme in the phase-two liver detoxification pathway. Women who had the NAT2 SNP and were smokers had a 2.4-fold risk of breast cancer.[6] Alcohol consumption has been linked with increased breast cancer in the past, but the mechanism has not been well understood. New research involving a polymorphism of the enzyme alcohol dehydrogenase may provide answers. Acetaldehyde, the first and most toxic metabolite of alcohol, is broken down by alcohol dehydrogenase (ADH) and aldehyde dehydrogenase (ALDH). Two separate studies have found that women with polymorphisms of these enzymes who drink even small amounts of alcohol have increased risk of breast cancer.[7,8] Other SNPs to consider in breast cancer are the enzymes that break down estrogens such as Cytochrome P450 1B1 and 3A4 and the methylation and glutathione pathway.

So which chemicals are linked to breast cancer?

Many chemicals in the environment are known to cause cancer and many chemicals are known to mimic estrogen in the body. I have chosen the most common chemicals women are exposed to in their everyday lives to highlight the link between chemicals and breast cancer.

The list includes:

♦ Polychlorinated Biphenols (PCBs)
♦ Polyaromatic Hydrocarbons (PAHs)
♦ Alcohol
♦ Dioxins
♦ Bisphenol-A (BPA)
♦ Pesticides
♦ Heterocyclic amines
♦ Phthalates
♦ Parabens
♦ Mercury
♦ Cadmium
♦ Lead

Polychlorinated Biphenols (PCBs) were used in electrical equipment and other products until the 1970s, when they were banned due to their cancer-causing effects. They remain in our soil and water today, and accumulate up the food chain. Our current source of exposure is through contaminated food. Researchers found women exposed to PCBs had a 2- to 4- fold increased risk of breast cancer, and the link was greater if the women had a genetic polymorphism of the CYP1A1 enzyme in the liver.[9] Women are exposed to PCBs without even knowing it due to their widespread presence in food and water.

Polyaromatic hydrocarbons (PAHs) are products of combustion found in auto exhaust, air pollution, tobacco smoke, and charbroiled meats. A high risk of breast cancer is associated with exposure to this carcinogen. The Long Island breast cancer study reported a 48% higher risk of breast cancer in women under 65 who had polyaromatic hydrocarbon-induced DNA damage in their blood than women without the polyaromatic-induced DNA damage.[10] This could mean that eating grilled meats and living in urban areas with high vehicle exhaust, which produce polyaromatic hydrocarbons, cause changes to the DNA, which leads to breast cancer.

Alcohol intake is linked to breast cancer as well. The connection between alcohol and breast cancer is an area of great controversy. The University of Cornell's Breast Cancer and Environmental Risk Factors program evaluated this issue in 1998 and released a fact sheet, which can be found at *http://envirocancer.cornell.edu/ factsheet/diet/fs13.alcohol.cfm.* Researchers there established that drinking 2 to 5 drinks per day is associated with a rate of breast cancer 40% greater than non-drinkers. The mechanism is thought to be that alcohol increases the level of estrogen in a woman's body.

Dioxins are formed by incineration, a method of disposing of waste through very high temperatures so it combusts. When certain waste materials, such as products made from polyvinyl chloride and polychlorinated biphenols, are incinerated, dioxins are released into the air. Dioxins pollute the air and waterways, contaminate feed and crops and eventually work their way into the food chain. Dioxins are a known cancer-causing agent according to the U.S. Environmental Protection Agency. Researchers have just begun to make the link between breast cancer and dioxins. Blood samples taken from women who were exposed to dioxins during an explosion in 1976 while working at a chemical plant in Italy, and they showed that those with high levels of dioxins had twice the risk of breast cancer of those without high levels of dioxins.[11] Women are exposed to low doses of dioxin through food and water.

Bisphenol-A (BPA) is a chemical found in hard plastic bottles, the lining of some metal food cans and some dental sealants. It was originally developed as a synthetic estrogen before it received approval to be used by the plastic industry. BPA is currently an area of controversy; some states are banning products that contain BPA while the industry and the FDA continue to state that it is safe. Studies in a lab using human breast cancer cells show that BPA stimulates breast cancer cell growth, just like human estrogen. [12] This makes sense, considering it was originally developed as a synthetic estrogen.

Pesticides have been in use in the U.S. since World War II. Today, most people use pesticides around their home to kill insects, bugs, fleas and rodents. Herbicides are applied to lawns, golf courses and parks to kill weeds. Insecticides are applied to pets to kill fleas. The agricultural industry uses the most pesticides, spraying crops, which can create residue on produce waiting to be sold at the store. Currently our air, water and soil are contaminated with pesticides. Even some pesticides, like DDT, that have been banned since the 1970s due to their carcinogenic effects, are still in our groundwater, rivers, lakes and oceans.

These pesticides accumulate throughout the food chain. Vegetables and fruits are grown in contaminated soil and watered with contaminated water. Animals eat feed contaminated with pesticides, and we eat the animals or their milk and eggs. Our air is polluted with pesticides from our neighbors spraying trying to kill weeds, or by the city dropping insecticides by plane to kill mosquitoes. Basically, they are everywhere. (Read chapter two on how we are exposed to chemicals.)

The question is: how are pesticides linked to breast cancer? Since cancer can take years to develop, it is interesting to look at the pesticide DDT, which has been banned since the 70s. A recent study measured blood levels of DDT in women when they were young and then tracked them over the next 20 to 25 years. They recorded whenever women were diagnosed with breast cancer before the age of 50 or died from breast cancer before the age of 50. The study concluded that exposure to DDT before the age of 14 was associated with a fivefold increase in risk of breast cancer before the age of 50.[13] What makes this study interesting is that many women exposed to DDT during adolescence in the early 1970s have yet to reach age 50. Does this mean we will see an increase in breast cancer in the next few years? It is difficult to answer this question, since cancer has many causes, takes years to develop, and involves many factors at play.

Studies in the laboratory that take breast cancer cells and add pesticides, such as DDT, show that pesticides have an estrogenic effect. Pesticides cause the breast cancer cells to grow and divide just like estrogen. This is significant since many breast cancer tumors are estrogen-receptor positive, meaning they react to estrogen stimulation. One study took 41 women undergoing breast biopsy for a mass in their breast and measured the level of pesticides in the breast tissue. Twenty of the women had breast cancer and 17 had benign disease and the others had dysplasia of the breast. The levels of DDT were higher in the women with breast cancer than those with benign disease, but what was more significant was that women with estrogen receptor (ER)-positive breast cancer had higher pesticide levels in the tissue than those with ER-negative breast cancer and without breast cancer.[14] These studies show that pesticides are estrogenic and that they are linked to health conditions that are mediated by estrogen, such as breast cancer.

A patient once asked me if she needed to be concerned about playing golf or spraying pesticides every now and then on her front lawn. Her thought was that it was such a low level of exposure and was something she did occasionally that it really wasn't a concern. I reminded her of Dr. William Rea's rain barrel analogy from Chapter Two. We are exposed every day to a little of this and a little of that, and over time these chemicals can build up in our body. These chemicals also may react with each other once in our body, and some people are good at clearing these chemicals through the liver while others are genetically set up to hang on to them. A report released in 2006 from the Long Island Breast Cancer Study Project showed that women, who reported using pesticides around the home, even occasionally, had an increased risk of breast cancer.[15]

Heterocyclic amines are formed from cooking meat at high temperatures. Any muscle meat from a cow, pig, chicken, turkey, or fish can produce these cancer-causing compounds when cooked at a high temperature. Women who ate well-done meat had 4.6-fold increased risk of breast cancer compared to women who ate rare or medium meat. The risk was correlated to levels of heterocyclic amines. Numerous animal studies have also linked heterocyclic amines from cooking meat to breast cancer.[16]

Phthalates are a group of chemicals added to plastics to make them soft and flexible. They are found in plastic bottles, plastic storage containers, plastic food wrap, polyvinyl chloride products such as plastic vinyl shower curtains and tablecloths, time-released medications, pesticides, cosmetics and many children's toys. Phthalates are known to disrupt women's reproductive hormones and are often called estrogen mimickers.[17]

We know from studies done on young girls who develop breasts at an early age that phthalates can influence breast cell growth, much like estrogen. A study done on young Puerto Rican girls with premature breast development showed that exposure to phthalates in the environment played a role in early breast growth.[18] Premature breast development and starting menses before age eight is called "precocious puberty."

Phthalates also directly stimulate the growth of breast cancer cells in the lab. Researchers often place breast cancer cells in a dish and add known environmental chemicals to watch for growth and stimulation of the cancer cells. This is how toxins are determined to be estrogenic, meaning they act like estrogen. Researchers also have determined that phthalates can interfere with the positive effects of a drug called tamoxifen, which is often given to women with breast cancer to increase their chances for survival and decrease recurrence.[19] The chapter on avoidance describes how to avoid phthalates in plastic.

Parabens are another group of chemicals that you are exposed to every day. They are in cosmetics, shampoos, lotions, soaps and many other grooming products. They are what keep bacteria from growing in the product. Common parabens used in cosmetic and grooming products are methylparaben, ethylparaben and propylparaben. Parabens are everywhere and in all of us. They have been found in women with breast cancer. More specifically, they have been found in the breast tumor. A 2004 study looked at a small sample of women with breast cancer and measured their tumor tissue for parabens. Each sample had parabens in it, with methylparaben the most frequently occurring.[20] Parabens act like estrogen in the body and can cause breast cancer cells in a lab to grow and proliferate.[21] It is important for women to use personal care products and cosmetics free of parabens.

Heavy metals (mercury, cadmium, lead)

These three metals are common in the environment. Mercury is in fish, which is probably the main source of exposure, and in our air. Cadmium is in cigarette smoke as well as contaminated soil, and thus in fruits and vegetables grown in that soil. Lead is in our air and water. (See glossary for more details on these metals.) Studies have shown that cadmium acts like estrogen in breast cancer cells by binding to the receptor.[22] The 2006 Journal of the National Cancer Institute, issue 12 page 869, published a study of 246 women with breast cancer and tested their urine for cadmium. Women with elevated urinary cadmium had twice the risk for breast cancer than age-matched controls. Lead and mercury also stimulate breast cancer cells and act like estrogen.[23] Studies have also found these metals in breast tissue taken from women with breast cancer as compared to breast tissue taken from women without breast cancer.[24]

Summary

So what does this all mean for women with breast cancer or women who want to prevent breast cancer? The exact cause of breast cancer remains unknown. We do know risk factors associated with breast cancer. The link to environmental chemicals is undeniable, but critics state more research needs to be done in this area. At what point will we stop researching and start regulating? Most of these chemicals are produced by industry and they end up in our food, air, water and products. As voters, consumers and patients, you have a voice; use it. Reading this book and discovering the links, following the guides on avoiding environmental toxins and then following the 8-week detoxification plan to remove what has already been stored in your body is a place to start.

Endometriosis

Endometriosis is a condition affecting 5% to 10% of women. The name comes from the word 'endometrium,' which is the tissue that lines the uterus. In a woman with endometriosis, this endometrial tissue is found outside of the uterus on the ovaries, fallopian tubes, and in the abdominal cavity. This tissue found outside of the uterus can respond to the menstrual cycle in the same way the lining of the uterus responds. At the end of the second half of the menstrual cycle, called the luteal phase, when hormones decline and the uterine lining is shed, endometrial tissue growing outside of the uterus will also break apart and bleed. This blood has no place to go so the surrounding tissue may become inflamed and swollen. This can cause pain and cramping. Scar tissue can form around the endometriosis sites and develop into areas called 'implants,' 'nodules,' 'lesions,' or 'growths.'[1] All of these terms are used interchangeably.

Endometriosis typically occurs in women of reproductive age, most commonly 25 to 30 years old at the time of diagnosis. However, in the past five years, I have seen this condition more and more in younger women, from age 15 to 25. Diagnosis is confirmed by laparoscopic surgery typically performed for complaints of pelvic pain or painful menstrual cycles. Endometriosis is a hormonally responsive condition. Endometriosis lesions contain estrogen, progesterone, and androgen receptors.[1] Risk of endometriosis seems related to the amount of menstrual flow. Women with a short menstrual cycle (less than 27days), longer menstrual flow (greater than 7days), and spotting before the onset of menses are at greater risk for developing endometriosis.[2] Endometriosis is found more commonly in Asian women than Caucasian women.[2]

The symptoms of endometriosis include:

♦ Painful menstrual periods
♦ Pelvic pain
♦ Pain with intercourse
♦ Lower abdominal pain or back pain
♦ Painful bowel movements (especially during menses)
♦ Painful urination (especially during menses)
♦ Pain with exercise
♦ Difficulty conceiving

Diagnosis can often be difficult and is sometimes delayed. Endometriosis is the underlying cause in 15% of pelvic pain cases, and it is also a common cause of infertility.[3] Endometriosis can adhere to the fallopian tubes and ovaries, affecting ovulation. The symptoms of endometriosis can mimic other conditions, which need to be ruled out. The gold standard for diagnosis is laparoscopy. Laparoscopy is a surgical procedure where a thin tube with a lens and a light is inserted into the abdomen through a small incision. The laparoscope allows the physician to see the pelvic area and locate endometrial growths. The laparoscope can also remove the endometriosis at the time of examination, thus offering treatment during diagnosis.

The exact cause and pathogenesis of endometriosis is unclear. Several theories exist, but none have been entirely proven. Many theories exist as to what causes endometriosis, and it is likely a combination of many factors that, together, not only determine the cause, but also the severity of the disease.

Possible causes of endometriosis:

♦ Retrograde menstruation – where the endometrial cells flow backwards through the fallopian tubes.

♦ Metaplasia – changing of one type of tissue to another.

♦ Genetic factors – women with first-degree relatives with endometriosis are predisposed to have the disease.

♦ Immunologic – inflammatory cytokines and autoimmune conditions.

♦ Iatrogenic – develops after pelvic surgery such as laproscopy, cesarean section, or hysterectomy.

♦ Nutrition – meat and dairy products.

♦ Environmental factors.

Environmental factors must be considered. Since endometriosis is a hormone responsive disease with an immunological component, environmental exposures that affect a woman's hormonal and immune system need to be addressed.

Such toxins include:

♦ Dioxins and Polychlorinated Biphenols (PCBs)
♦ Phthalates
♦ Bisphenol-A
♦ Pesticides
♦ Solvents
♦ Formaldehyde
♦ Heavy metal-cadmium

Dioxins and PCBs are organochlorine compounds that contaminate our food and water, and women are often exposed to low doses on a daily basis. Deep endometriotic nodules in women with endometriosis are associated with high blood levels of dioxin and PCBs.[4]

Phthalates are used in the plastic industry and are in everything from plastic water bottles with "#3" on the bottom to plastic cling wrap to cosmetics. A recent study of 55 women with endometriosis showed that women with endometriosis had higher blood levels of phthalates compared to 55 women without endometriosis.[5] Women in the United States are not the only ones suffering from the effects of chemicals in the environment. A study published in the British Journal of Obstetrics and Gynecology in 2006 looked at 49 women in India who were infertile due to endometriosis and compared them to 38 women who were infertile due to some other cause, such as pelvic inflammatory disease and fibroids, and found that the women with endometriosis had higher levels of phthalates in their blood than women without endometriosis.[6]

Bisphenol-A is a known estrogen mimicker and is present in the lining of metal food cans and plastic bottles. A study done comparing women with endometriosis to healthy women found that over 63% of the women with endometriosis had BPA in their blood, and none of the healthy women had BPA in their blood. This study, of course, only shows a correlation, and doesn't necessarily mean that BPA caused the endometriosis. But given the fact that BPA is a known hormone disrupting chemical and is found in many consumer products, women with endometriosis should consider avoiding this source of exposure.[7]

Pesticides and insecticides, which are often used around homes, at parks and on golf courses, have been shown to either be directly estrogenic or have estrogenic contaminants and could affect the growth of endometriosis implants. Even pesticides that are no longer used in this country but are still in the soil and waterways are linked to endometriosis.[8] As mentioned in Chapter Two, pesticides in the soil and waterways can accumulate up the food chain and contaminate farmed fish and meats.

Formaldehyde and solvents are chemicals present in furniture, wood, carpet, upholstery, dry-cleaning, household cleaners, and many other products. You are exposed through air, water and absorption through the skin. One study looked at high-dose exposure, such as women working in the wood-making industry and laboratory workers, and found a connection to endometriosis.[9]

Cadmium is a heavy metal present in cigarette smoke, including secondhand smoke, shellfish, green leafy vegetables, and food grown using soil or water contaminated with cadmium. Using data from the National Health and Nutrition Examination Survey, researchers found that women with endometriosis had higher blood levels of cadmium than women without endometriosis.[10]

Summary

It is always difficult to say that just because something in high doses causes endometriosis, it will do the same in low doses. I just keep in mind the rain barrel analogy. You are exposed every day to a little bit of this chemical plus a little bit of that chemical, which over time, builds up in your body, mixes together and, unless it is removed, will eventually cause disease and illness.

Most women are exposed to environmental toxins on some level every day. However, not all women get endometriosis. Some women are genetically set up to have trouble clearing hormones such as estrogen and environmental estrogens through their body. Single nucleotide polymorphisms (SNPs) might provide an explanation as to why some women clear exposures easily and others do not, making them more susceptible to the hormone disrupting effects. SNP is a genetic change in which a single base in the DNA is altered. This simple change can affect how our bodies detoxify environmental toxins. Since most toxins are cleared through the liver, it is important to look at what SNPs in the liver are associated with endometriosis. Recent studies have shown that women with a polymorphism of the cytochrome P450 1A1 gene and the glutathione S-tranferase M1 gene have increased risk of endometriosis.[11] In the testing chapter of this book, I will explain polymorphisms in greater detail and discuss simple methods for testing for SNPs. Some women seem to have difficulty clearing toxins through their liver. This means that, all other things being equal, they would be the ones to accumulate the highest level of toxins in their body. As it turns out, these slow detoxifiers also have an increased risk of endometriosis. This is another clue that environmental toxins may be behind endometriosis.

Fibroids of the Uterus

Many women develop small tumors inside the uterus. These are called "leiomyomas" or "fibroids." These growths are not actually made of fibrous material, but of uterine smooth-muscle cells and connective tissue. Fibroids form from genetically abnormal cells in the wall of the uterus. The cells are non-cancerous, or benign, and their growth is believed to be stimulated by estrogen. Some studies have suggested that fibroids have a higher number of estrogen receptors in the fibroid tissue than normal uterine wall tissue.[1] Fibroid growth is typically regulated by estrogen, and fibroids grow during pregnancy when hormones rise, and regress after menopause when hormones decline.

There are three main types of uterine fibroids: Subserosal, which grow from the outer wall of the uterus; intramural, which grow from within the uterine wall muscle; and submucosal, which grow from just under the uterine tissue. Fibroids vary in size ranging from smaller growth, about 1 cm, to very large growths, up to 10 cm. They may or may not cause symptoms; however, fibroids are the reason most women end up getting a hysterectomy. They account for one-third of all hysterectomies in the U.S. Most fibroids are diagnosed with a pelvic ultrasound and, depending on the size and location, can be felt by your doctor during a pelvic exam.

Symptoms of fibroids may include:

◆ Pressure in the abdomen;
◆ Pelvic pain
◆ Heavy menstrual bleeding
◆ Spotting
◆ Infertility
◆ Miscarriage
◆ Urinary symptoms
◆ Uterine enlargement

♦ Pain with intercourse
♦ Backache

The reason fibroids grow inside the uterus remains unknown, but risk factors include starting your menses at a young age, never having children, being overweight, age, using birth control pills with certain kinds of hormones, hormone replacement therapy in menopause, genetics, and, of course, environmental causes such as environmental estrogen mimickers.[2] When you look at the list of possible causes, the main theme is the hormone estrogen. This is why, if a woman has fibroids that are not causing any problems and she is very close to menopause, most physicians will leave them alone, because once a woman goes into menopause, the fibroids typically shrink.

Many chemicals in the environment act like estrogen in the body. Since fibroids are estrogen-stimulated, one must consider environmental factors as either an initiator or a promoter of these benign growths. Common chemicals present in our food, air and water—which we are exposed to in small doses every day—may contribute to the growth of fibroids.

Chemicals linked to fibroids include:

♦ Pesticides
♦ Polychlorinated biphenols
♦ Dioxins
♦ Phthalates
♦ Heavy metals

Pesticides and Polychlorinated Biphenols (PCBs) are chemicals we are exposed to every day, even though some pesticides, such as DDT and PCBs, have been banned in the U.S. We are still exposed through farmed fish and some meat products and well as through in-utero exposure when a mother has a high body burden of chemicals and passes them to the unborn child through the placental barrier. Numerous studies have linked low doses of these chemicals to fibroids.

Here are the highlights:

♦ Women with fibroids had higher blood levels of the pesticide **DDT** than women without fibroids.

♦ Higher levels of **DDT** and its metabolite **DDE** were found in the tissue of fibroids than in normal myometrium.[1]

♦ In a study of 489 women, high blood levels of **PCBs** and **pesticides** were found in women with fibroids and endometriosis.[3]

♦ The pesticide **methoxychlor**, which is commonly used in the U.S., was found to increase fibroid cell growth as well as a pesticide called **keptone**, which was banned in the U.S. because of its estrogenic activity.[4] Although keptone was banned, it is still present in our rivers, lakes and soil and is a contaminant in food.

Dioxins are the name for a group of hundreds of chemicals that are present everywhere in the environment. The most toxic compound is 2,3,7,8-tetrachlorodibenzo-p-dioxin, or TCDD. Dioxin does not naturally exist in the environment. It is formed as a byproduct of industrial processes involving chlorine, such as waste incineration, chemical and pesticide manufacturing and paper bleaching. Dioxin was the primary toxic component of Agent Orange. The main way we are currently exposed to dioxins is through our food and chlorinated herbicides, which are commonly used by many golf courses. It is a contaminant in meat, dairy and fish. Dioxins have been proven to be estrogenic, but studies linking them to uterine fibroids have been inconsistent. As mentioned earlier in the book, in 1976, there was a chemical explosion in Seveso, Italy. Women who were exposed had their blood taken soon after the explosion and tested for the dioxin TCDD; they had the highest documented levels in a human population. Researchers tracked 956 of the women for 20 years and found that 26.3% developed fibroids. The study found that the women who developed fibroids had low levels of TCDD in their blood, actually showing an anti-estrogenic effect of TCDD.[5]

Phthalates are continuously being examined for their estrogenic effects and links to reproductive problems in humans. Only in the past five years have researchers begun to explore the link to fibroids. There are only a few studies on phthalates and fibroids, and most only date back 4 or 5 years. However, from 1999 to 2002, the National Health and Nutrition Examination Survey (NHANES) took place in the U.S. It was designed to represent the average U.S. citizen. An analysis from NHANES looked at 947 women who had their urinary levels of phthalates collected. The study revealed that women with fibroids had high levels of a common phthalate metabolite called mono-n-butyl phthalate (MnBP).[6] MnBP is a breakdown product or metabolite of the chemical di-n-butyl phthalate, which is added to plastics, paint, glue, hairspray, and other household products. It is commonly found in the environment, and most people are exposed to low levels in the air, water, and food.

Cadmium is a heavy metal that we are all exposed to in low doses every day through the air, our food and our water. In a study of 501 women whose body burden of heavy metals was determined through a urine heavy metal test, a correlation was found between cadmium and uterine fibroids.[7] The heavy metal test was administered by giving the women 10mg/kg of 2,3,-dimercaptropropane-1-sulfonic acid (DMPS) followed by a urine collection at 2 hours and then 3 hours after taking the DMPS. This type of heavy metal test is called a provocative test or challenge test because the DMPS will bind metals from storage sites in the body, giving a more accurate picture of total load of metals in the body than a simple blood test.

This test can be administered with oral or intravenous DMPS, oral DMSA or intravenous EDTA. You can read more on heavy metal testing in the chapter on testing for toxins.

Mercury and lead are two other common heavy metals that we come into contact with on a daily basis. Mercury is found in fish, herbicides, wood preservatives, antiseptics, thermometers and dental fillings. Lead is found in paint, printed material, fuels, pottery, and drinking water. The National Health and Nutrition Examination Survey found a link between high serum levels of mercury, lead and uterine fibroids.[8]

Summary

Uterine fibroids are considered to be an estrogen-dependent condition that affects numerous women and is often the reason women get hysterectomies. Uterine fibroid tissue has been found to express estrogen receptors. This is why environmental estrogens need to be considered when deciding the best approach to treatment. In clinical practice, I have found that by taking an in-depth environmental exposure history, knowing which toxins are linked to fibroids and testing for those chemicals helps guide my treatment. Treatment is aimed at removing chemicals from the body with an 8-week detoxification plan, increasing estrogen clearance in the liver, and education on avoiding environmental estrogen.

Fibromyalgia, Chronic Fatigue, Chemical Sensitivity

Fibromyalgia syndrome (FMS), chronic fatigue syndrome (CFS), and multiple chemical sensitivity (MCS) is an increasingly common group of syndromes that tend to affect women more than men. They are classified as syndromes and are diagnosed based on a set of symptoms. Fibromyalgia is a chronic condition characterized by generalized pain throughout the body, specific trigger points, fatigue (often chronic fatigue), and sleep disturbances. Persons with fibromyalgia and chronic fatigue tend to be more sensitive to exposure to chemicals and odors from chemicals. This is called multiple chemical sensitivity or chemical intolerance.

Multiple chemical sensitivity (MCS) is a condition in which a person experiences negative health effects in many organ systems from exposure to low levels of common chemicals. Exposure can be from inhalation, such as breathing in someone else's perfume, or from absorption through the skin, such as coming into contact with a cleaning product or detergent, or from ingestion, such as eating or drinking something with heavy metal or pesticide contamination. There has been some progress made in the development of a standard definition for MCS, but mostly the diagnosis is based on symptoms.

People with MCS suffer from intolerance to low levels of chemicals in the environment. They experience negative health effects in response to chemicals. The effects may range from mild to severe and can include fibromyalgia and chronic fatigue.

Common symptoms include:

- Headache
- Dizziness
- Nausea
- Musculoskeletal pain-fibromyalgia syndrome
- Poor memory and concentration
- Depression, anxiety
- Irritability
- Fatigue-chronic fatigue syndrome
- Digestive disturbances
- Skin rashes

There is still much debate as to what causes these three conditions or syndromes. One study showed a link to low magnesium and zinc levels.[1] Other theories include genetics, physical trauma, or an infection with a bacteria or virus as an initiator of fibromyalgia. What is known is that all three of these syndromes have overlapping physiological effects in the body, risk factors, and treatments.[2]

The question that remains to be answered is this: Can chemicals in the environment initiate these conditions? There isn't much research in this area, but clinically I see that most of my patients with MCS, fibromyalgia and chronic fatigue have high levels of either lead or mercury in their bodies and, with chelation and cleansing, most of their symptoms improve. Most of these patients have a significant exposure history as well. One patient of mine had had symptoms of fibromyalgia and chronic fatigue for five years. She came to see me for naturopathic treatment. During the intake she mentioned that she was also sensitive to chemicals and avoided the detergent aisle at the grocery store. When she was around detergents and perfumes she would get a headache and have trouble breathing. I took an in-depth environmental exposure history and discovered that while she was in engineering school, she'd had exposure to solvents while in the organic chemistry lab. She was also a teaching assistant for the lab for one year. I ran some simple tests for environmental chemicals, and a urine solvent panel showed elevated levels of solvents in her body. I treated her for solvent exposure by having her undergo a cleansing and detoxification program similar to what is outlined in the treatment section of this book. After three months of treatment, her symptoms improved by 80%.

One 1998 study looked at chemical initiators of fibromyalgia, chronic fatigue, and chemical sensitivity and found that volatile organic compounds played a role. The study showed that exposure to these chemicals that was at high doses initially, and then at lower doses later, seemed to trigger fibromyalgia, chronic fatigue or chemical sensitivity.[3]

Volatile organic compounds include:

♦ Solvents
♦ Formaldehyde
♦ Heavy metals
♦ Pesticides

Let's look at other environmental links

Organochlorine compounds are a class of chemicals that includes pesticides, dioxins, PCBs, polyvinyl chloride products, and more. The best known organochloride is the pesticide DDT. We know that DDT is linked to chronic fatigue from studies done comparing patients with chronic fatigue to healthy controls. The patients with chronic fatigue had higher levels of DDT in their blood.[4]

In a 1997 review of chemical exposures and fibromyalgia, chronic fatigue, and multiple chemical sensitivity, the link is made clear. The study is a review of all the evidence up to 1997. Clearly there is more recent research, the fact that the link was made back in 1997 and these conditions are still not recognized by conventional physicians demonstrates why it is often difficult for patients to get properly diagnosed and treated.[5]

Chemical sensitivity has been reported following exposure to:

♦ Chlordane
♦ Chlorpyrifos
♦ Pesticides
♦ Formaldehyde
♦ Solvents in cleaning products
♦ Chloroform from swimming in a pool

67% of patients with fibromyalgia and chronic fatigue reported that their symptoms worsened upon exposure to:[5]

♦ Gas
♦ Paint
♦ Solvent fumes

Summary

As new research emerges, perhaps we will get a better understanding of fibromyalgia syndrome, chronic fatigue syndrome and multiple chemical sensitivity. It is important to remember that symptoms of the three syndromes typically appear together in a person who is affected. Often a chemical exposure initiates the syndromes, or some other cause is present and chemical exposure merely exacerbates the symptoms. Whatever the case, there is hope for treatment.

Heart Disease

Cardiovascular diseases (CVD) are the number one leading cause of death in the United States, according to the American Heart Association. The terms "cardiovascular disease" and "heart disease" are often used interchangeably and could mean someone suffers from atherosclerosis, hypertension, arrhythmias, congenital heart defects, and more. Although many people think of heart disease as a man's problem, women can and do get heart disease. In fact, heart disease is the number one killer of women in the United States. It is also a leading cause of disability among women. The older a woman gets, the more likely she is to get heart disease. But women of all ages should be concerned about heart disease. All women can take steps to prevent it by practicing a healthy lifestyle and considering environmental toxins.

Risk factors for heart disease include:

♦ Congenital heart defects
♦ Coronary artery disease
♦ High blood pressure
♦ Diabetes
♦ Smoking
♦ Excessive use of alcohol or caffeine
♦ Drug abuse
♦ Stress
♦ Obesity
♦ Poor nutrition
♦ Over-the-counter medications and prescription medications
♦ Genetic polymorphisms
♦ Environmental toxins

Chemicals such as heavy metals, solvents, bisphenol-A, and others have been linked to heart disease. We are exposed to these through air pollution, drinking water, cigarette smoke, plastics, and food. These toxins play a role in the initiation or progression of heart disease. They affect the heart by causing inflammation, atherosclerosis, affecting aortic smooth muscle cells, oxidative metabolism, phospholipid turnover, and protein and enzyme function in the heart and vessels.[1]

Toxins to consider:

♦ Heavy metals
♦ Bisphenol-A
♦ Solvents
♦ Air pollution
♦ Particulate matter

Lead and high blood pressure: Numerous studies have shown an association between low-dose exposure to lead and hypertension.[2] Elevated blood pressure is a leading risk factor for cardiovascular disease morbidity and mortality in the U.S. Lead may affect blood pressure indirectly by affecting kidney function and the rennin-angiotensin system.[3] Most people are exposed to lead through contaminated drinking water from old lead pipes, contaminated food from improperly glazed ceramic dishes, air pollution, hair dyes, cosmetics and hobbies. Recent exposure to lead may be circulating in the blood; however, most lead is eventually stored in the bone. In postmenopausal women who start to lose bone density and develop osteopenia, stored lead may be released back into the blood, causing increased blood pressure and heart disease.[3]

Lead: The Journal of the American Heart Association, called *Circulation*, released a study in 2006 showing that low levels of lead in the blood are linked to an increase in cardiovascular mortality. This study was significant because the link was found at blood levels much lower than previously studied.

Mercury: Methylmercury exposure through fish consumption may increase the risk of cardiovascular disease. The heart is one of the target organs of mercury and can affect heart development in the womb as well as the cardiac sodium channel, can block Na-K-ATPase, can cause atherosclerosis, and can damage lipids in the blood or lipid peroxidation. In one study, fish intake and subsequent hair mercury levels were correlated with increased risk of heart attack and cardiovascular disease.[4] Several factors are likely to be at play in determining cardiovascular risk from mercury. The beneficial omega-3 fatty acids in fish have heart protective effects, but excessive mercury exposure is likely to outweigh those beneficial effects.

Cadmium: Elevated cadmium levels in the blood are associated with high blood pressure. One study looked at low levels of cadmium exposure in non-smokers and found increased risk of mild hypertension.[5] Diet and air pollution are the main sources of exposure to low levels of cadmium in the general population. Smoking and secondhand smoke are also major sources of exposure.

Arsenic is a metal that most people are exposed to through drinking water, food (especially chicken), pesticides, wood used to construct decks and playgrounds, and some medications and glass. Arsenic is a risk factor for atherosclerosis, coronary disease and stroke. The mechanism is not exactly known, although arsenic can cause an increase in reactive oxygen species, lipid peroxidation, can up regulate inflammatory signals, and can induce atherosclerosis.[5]

Bisphenol-A (BPA) is found in plastic beverage bottles, the lining of food cans and dental sealants. We are exposed to Bisphenol-A at low doses every day. Besides having reproductive effects in men and women, it also can cause cardiovascular disease. High urine level of BPA is associated with angina, MI, coronary heart disease, and alterations in lipids and liver enzymes.[6]

Solvents are found in hair dye, paints, cosmetics, cleaning products, industrial chemicals, dry-cleaning, gasoline, and many other products. We use solvents in our everyday lives without realizing we may be absorbing them through the skin or inhaling the fumes. Solvents are known to cause heart arrhythmias. Toluene from paint, benzene from cigarette smoke and auto exhaust, and chloroform and trichloroethylene from the shower, are among the many solvents that can cause cardiac arrhythmias.[7]

Air pollution is composed of a mixture of chemicals and substances such as heavy metals, solvents, polycyclic hydrocarbons, pesticides, ozone, and particulate matter. These chemicals come from many sources, such as dust, auto exhaust, jet fuel, pesticide spraying, industry, trash incineration, coal-burning power plants and more. This makes it difficult to separate one pollutant's effects from the other. Air pollution has been linked to increased risk of hypertension, stroke, inflammation, acute heart attack, deep vein thrombosis (blood clot) and atherosclerosis.[8]

Particulate matter (PM) is a mixture of small particles and liquid droplets. It is composed of acids (such as nitrates and sulfates), organic chemicals, metals, and soil or dust particles. The size of particles is important in determining if PM has an effect on health. The EPA is concerned about particles that are 10 micrometers in diameter or smaller. These pass through the throat and nose and enter the lungs. Once inhaled, these particles can affect the heart and lungs and cause serious health effects. Find more information at *www.epa.gov/particles/*.

Particulate matter that is inhaled into the lungs causes oxidative stress, which leads to systemic inflammation that can increase cardiovascular disease. This occurs through thickening of the blood or development of atherosclerotic plaques.[9]

Summary

There are numerous risk factors for the development of cardiovascular disease. In managing cardiovascular disease or when working on prevention of heart disease, environmental factors cannot be ignored. Education on avoidance of toxins is the first step in prevention and treatment. Low-dose exposure to environmental toxins through the air, water, food, and products has not received much attention in the past. They are directly linked to heart disease. Attention to these environmental risk factors, educating each other, creating health-protective public policies, and modifying our behavior at home and at work is likely to decrease cardiovascular disease in the U.S.

Infertility

If you have been trying to conceive without success, you are not alone. More than 1 out of 10 couples in the U.S. have trouble conceiving. Infertility is defined as an inability to conceive after one year of unprotected intercourse. Some sources define infertility more specifically as having unprotected intercourse one to three times a week for one year and failing to get pregnant. Trouble conceiving can put strain on a relationship, can be the source of heartache, and can lead to stress and unexpected medical expenses. Typically at some point in trying to get pregnant, couples turn to their physician for answers.

Many factors account for infertility in men and women. One medical source, *http://www.multicare-assoc.com/health/infertility. asp*, states that male causes of infertility account for roughly 35% of the problem, and female factors are the issue 65% of the time. Of course, there are factors that affect both men and women such as age, obesity, alcohol, cigarettes, drugs, cancer and its treatments, medical conditions such as thyroid disorders, Cushing's syndrome, diabetes, and kidney disease, and, of course, environmental factors.[1]

Male fertility problems include:

♦ Abnormal sperm production or function, including:
♦ Impaired sperm shape and movement
♦ Absent production in the testicles
♦ Low sperm count
♦ Varicolcele
♦ Undescended testicle
♦ Genetic disorders
♦ Testosterone deficiency

Impaired delivery of sperm, including:

♦ Erectile dysfunction
♦ Retrograde ejaculation
♦ No semen
♦ Blockage of ducts
♦ Hypospadias
♦ Anti-sperm antibodies

Female fertility problems include:

♦ Fallopian tube damage or blockage, including:
♦ Pelvic inflammatory disease
♦ Endometriosis
♦ Adhesions

Ovulatory and hormonal disorders, including:

♦ Polycystic ovarian syndrome
♦ Premature ovarian failure
♦ Luteal phase defect
♦ Hyperprolactinemia

Cervical, uterine problems, including:

♦ Fibroids
♦ Polyps
♦ Stenosis

Once couples realize they are having trouble conceiving, they may seek medical care. This involves a full medical work-up of both the man and the woman, and often leads to a visit to a reproductive specialist. This is where fertility care and treatment in the U.S. starts to get expensive. Fertility testing and treatment can run into the tens of thousands of dollars, and is often not covered by insurance. Often, a cause is discovered and treatment is begun and pregnancy is achieved. Sometimes infertility goes unexplained, a cause is not discovered and fertility treatments fail. We should step back and ask why this is. What causes some of the problems with women's hormones that lead to infertility, and what causes some of the problems with males' sperm, testicles and penises that lead to infertility? This is where environmental toxins may provide the missing link.

Although infertility can be caused by many different factors, a significant portion of them are unexplained. Many suggest that environmental factors play a role. We know that low-dose exposure to chemicals in the environment alter male and female hormones and affect reproductive organs and glands. An organization called The Collaborative on Health and the Environment wrote a report summarizing the outcomes of the Women's Reproductive Health and Environmental Workshop, held in January 2008 in Bolinas, California. The report outlines which toxins are linked to infertility, and it can be found at *http://www.healthandenvironment.org/articles/doc/5492*.

The short list from the report includes:

♦ Pesticide DDT and its metabolite DDE
♦ Bispehnol-A
♦ Cigarette smoke
♦ Polychlorinated biphenols

Let's look more in-depth at some of these and highlight other common chemicals we come into contact with every day in small amounts through our food, air, water and products.

These chemicals are known to cause infertility:

Cigarette smoke is by itself an environmental toxin. It contains heavy metals, solvents, pesticides, and formaldehyde among its 4,000 chemical constituents. Men and women are exposed to cigarette smoke through active and passive smoking. Secondhand smoke is considered passive smoking. The link to infertility was discovered in 1983 when a study linked decreased fertility in couples to smoking cigarettes.[2] A review of 12 studies published between 1985 and 1997 linked infertility in women to smoking cigarettes.[2] Women experiencing infertility and who were undergoing expensive fertility procedures such as egg retrieval and in-vitro fertilization had poor outcomes if they were smokers.[2] Studies involving male infertility also found a link between smoking and poor sperm count, sperm motility and sperm size and shape.[2]

Lindane is a commonly used insecticide used on humans to treat scabies and lice. Studies have shown that lindane interacts with sperm and affects its lipid bi-layer. It also may inhibit sperm's response to female hormones in the uterus at the site of egg fertilization.[3]

Pentachlorophenol is a chemical used as a pesticide and as a wood preservative. It is no longer available to the general public. It is still used industrially as a wood preservative for utility poles, railroad ties, and wharf pilings. It is found in the air, water and soil and can be in our fish and other foods. This chemical can cause hormonal effects in a woman, leading to a decrease in ovarian and adrenal function, which can lead to infertility.[3]

Polychlorinated Biphenols (PCBs) once used in electrical equipment, plasticizers and adhesives, have now contaminated our fish, meats and dairy products. PCBs decrease fertility by lowering progesterone levels and altering estrogen and the ovulatory cycle.[4]

Chlorinated hydrocarbons were found in the blood of 489 women struggling with infertility.[4] Chlorinated hydrocarbons are a group of chemicals that include pesticides such as DDT, solvents such as chloroform, polyvinyl chloride products, and others. They are known to alter the hypothalamic-pituitary-ovarian axis, which regulates the menstrual cycle and ovulation. These chemicals also alter estrogen and progesterone in a woman and directly affect the maturing egg as it comes from the ovary.[5]

Perfluorooctane sulfonate (PFOS) and perfluorooctanoate (PFOA) are chemicals that belong to a class called perfluorinated chemicals (PFCs). These are used in clothing, firefighting foams, carpet, furniture, and personal care products. They have contaminated our soil, water, and air. PFCs have accumulated up the food chain and are present in food as well as products. In a study published in 2009 in the journal called Human Reproduction, PFOS and PFOA were associated with longer waits before achieving pregnancy.[6] Blood levels of these chemicals were elevated in women with menstrual irregularities, longer wait times before pregnancy, and increased odds of infertility.

Fish consumption and mercury levels are also linked to infertility. We know from government health warnings that certain fish contain high levels of mercury. (See Chapter Two for a list of fish high in mercury). The advisories are typically aimed at women who are pregnant or breast feeding, and advise them to avoid fish high in mercury due to its toxic effects on pregnancy and developing newborns. But what about the general public's consumption of fish high in mercury? Are there any health effects or any links to infertility? One study of infertile couples found that couples who were infertile had high blood levels of circulating mercury compared to couples who were not infertile. It went on to directly correlate the high mercury levels and fish consumption. The more fish the infertile couples ate, the higher levels of mercury in their blood.[7]

Don't forget the men

Although this is a women's health book, infertility involves both men and women. There is a growing awareness around the effects of chemicals in the environment on fertility in both men and women. Much research has been done looking at the hormone mimicking and hormone altering effects of these chemicals. Now studies are looking at the effects on sperm as well. In Western countries, sperm counts have declined by half during the past 50 years. In Denmark, up to 10% of men have sperm counts in the infertile range and 30% in the sub-fertile range. Again, chemicals are linked to hormonal changes in men and direct toxic insult on the testicles, penis and sperm itself.[8,9,10]

Male factor environmental links:

♦ Mercury
♦ Phthalates
♦ Pesticides
♦ Cigarette smoke
♦ Organochlorines
♦ Bisphenol-A
♦ Dioxins

Summary

Infertility can be emotionally and physically draining on a woman and on a couple. Many factors are at play. Considering environmental factors that disrupt hormones may be the missing link. The modern day woman is exposed to more chemicals in her daily life than has ever been true before. It is important to take steps to avoid those chemicals, learn which specific chemicals are linked to infertility and begin to cleanse and detoxify the body.

Miscarriage and Premature Birth

Pregnancy is a time in a woman's life that is filled with many emotions, including excitement about the future, hormonal influences on mood, anticipation, and fear of something going wrong. The thought of losing the pregnancy is one of these fears. Although most pregnancies progress normally, some end in miscarriage. The medical term for miscarriage is spontaneous abortion, and this refers to the loss of pregnancy before the fetus is developed enough to survive on its own. In the scientific literature, miscarriage is defined as the loss of pregnancy before the twentieth week, although more than 80% of the time it happens in the first trimester.

Half of miscarriages are caused by chromosomal or structural abnormalities. Other known causes of miscarriage include infections, immune system abnormalities and hormonal irregularities. An OB/GYN typically identifies these causes during a thorough evaluation. The older a woman is, the more likely she will miscarry. Women between the ages of 35 and 40 have around a 14% chance of miscarriage, and women over 40 have about a 23% chance of miscarriage. This is in part due to chromosomal abnormalities that increase with age. Heavy cigarette smoking and alcohol consumption in both men and women increases the risk of miscarriage.[1] About one-third of miscarriages have no known cause.

Scientists suggest that environmental factors also influence pregnancy. Our environment is burdened with chemicals that are in the products we use daily, our food, water, air, and soil. There is a strong association between miscarriage and chemicals such as heavy metals, solvents, phthalates, polychlorinated biphenyls and pesticides, just to name a few.

Chemicals linked to miscarriage include:

Heavy metals: Low to moderate lead exposure may increase the risk for miscarriage.[2,3] Lead is a heavy metal that can be found in contaminated drinking water, old lead-based paint, leaded gas, newsprint and colored ads, hair dyes and rinses, pesticides, pencils, fertilizers, tobacco smoke, cosmetics, and ceramics. Other heavy metals linked to miscarriage include mercury and cadmium.[4] Women are exposed to mercury through petroleum products, fungicides, cosmetics, hair dyes, thermometers, vaccinations, silver dental fillings and consumption of saltwater fish. Common cadmium sources include cigarette smoke, contaminated drinking water, paints, welding, and shellfish.

Solvents are a variety of chemicals used in dry-cleaning, auto repair, paints, glues, gasoline, electronics, health care products, and household cleaning products. Toluene, xylene, and styrene are solvents commonly found in these sources, and all have been linked to miscarriage.[5] Solvents found in hair dyes, permanent solutions and dry-cleaning have also been linked to miscarriage.[1,5]

Phthalates are chemicals added to plastics to make them soft, strong and flexible. They are used in the manufacture of automotive parts, plastic wrap and storage containers, the lining of metal cans, medications, supplements, and some grooming products. Several studies link phthalates to hormone disrupting conditions in women, and they are linked to miscarriages in rats.[5]

Polychlorinated biphenyl (PCB) and pesticide exposure increases the risk for miscarriage.[1, 5, 6, 7] PCBs were once used in electrical transformers, capacitors, plasticizers and adhesives. Although many are no longer used in the U.S., they still persist in the environment. Fish from contaminated waters and farm raised fish, are major sources of PCBs, as are dairy and meat products. Pesticides are widely used in agriculture and home lawn care. Some have been banned due to their toxic side effects but these too persist in the environment today. Our major source of exposure is pesticide residue on non-organic fruits and vegetables.

Bisphenol-A is another common chemical that we are exposed to every day through the lining of metal food cans, dental sealants and plastic bottles. A recent study linked blood levels of BPA to repeated miscarriage. The study examined 45 women with a history of three or more consecutive first-trimester miscarriages and compared them to healthy women. The women who had experienced repeated miscarriage had higher levels of BPA in their body than the other women. This link is important, since we are exposed to BPA every day. BPA binds to estrogen receptors in the body and has 0.00025 times the estrogenic activity of the human estrogen estradiol.[8]

Women are exposed to these compounds every day. It is clear that environmental factors need to be evaluated when the cause of miscarriage is unknown. Some may argue that environmental toxins can account for some of the known causes of miscarriage, such as chromosomal, immune and hormonal abnormalities. Regardless, a thorough environmental evaluation should be considered.

Preterm birth

Since miscarriage is technically defined as loss of pregnancy before the twentieth week, we define pregnancies that almost make it to term as premature or preterm. Rates of preterm birth have been rising over the past several decades. Preterm birth is also linked to toxins in the environment. Recently, it was found that over 1,000 women who gave birth prematurely were three times more likely to have high blood levels of mercury. Even more interesting is that the mercury exposure was linked to fish consumption. Women who ate more fish had higher mercury levels and were more likely to give birth early.[9] Another study on preterm birth found that women who gave birth prematurely had high third-trimester urinary levels of phthalates compared to controls. Phthalates are prevalent in our environment, are estrogenic, and are linked to numerous hormonal conditions in women.[10]

Summary

There is evidence linking high-risk occupations to miscarriage and premature birth, but I wanted to highlight low-dose exposure to chemicals and these conditions. The balancing of a woman's hormonal system is a very delicate and complicated process. In pregnancy, it is critical. So many chemicals in our environment have the potential to act like hormones in the body and disrupt this delicate balance. Understanding which chemicals we come into contact with every day and have the potential to act as hormone mimickers or disruptors is key to a healthy pregnancy. A physician experienced in environmental medicine can test for these compounds in the blood and body tissues. If testing reveals that toxic compounds are present in the body, a comprehensive cleansing protocol can be designed by an experienced physician. Pharmaceutical agents are available to bind heavy metals and remove them from the body. Specific vitamins, minerals, herbs and amino acids are known to assist the body in detoxifying pesticides, solvents and other chemicals. These will be discussed in later chapters.

Osteoporosis

Osteoporosis is a thinning of bone tissue and loss of bone density that happens with aging. Bone health is critically important in aging for overall health and quality of life. Healthy bones provide the body with a frame that allows for mobility and for protection against injury. Bones serve as a storehouse for minerals that are vital to the functioning of many other systems in the body. Thin bones can lead to debilitating fractures and poor health. Osteoporotic fractures are a major cause of morbidity (illness) and mortality (death). Osteoporosis mostly affects women after menopause but can strike at any time and can affect men as well. A number of risk factors for developing osteoporosis have been identified.

Osteoporosis risk factors include:

- Age
- Being female
- Body size (thin)
- Years of estrogen deficiency
- Family history
- Low calcium intake and other nutrient deficiencies
- Smoking/alcohol
- Medical conditions
- Medications such as prednisone
- Fair skin/blond hair

Some may argue that having osteoporosis is not by itself an indicator of poor health or quality of life. What is more important is risk of a bone fracture. If a woman with thin bones falls and sustains a fracture, then she is more likely to have health complications than a woman with healthy bones is. So what causes someone to fracture a bone as they age?

Known risk factors for fractures include:

- Decreased bone mass/low bone density
- Age
- History of falling
- Previous fractures

When someone falls, that person won't necessarily sustain a bone fracture. However, if the bones are thin, it is more likely that a fall will result in a fracture. I used to be an occupational therapist working with patients in skilled nursing facilities. I can't tell you how many times I have seen a healthy, independent older person fall, sustain a fracture and end up needing rehab. In rehab, the goal is always to get people back to independent living, but often they end up needing assistance. This is how osteoporosis affects quality of life, and why osteoporosis prevention is critical for both men and women as we age.

So what exactly causes loss of bone density or thinning of the bones? In women, the loss of estrogen plays a key role. As estrogen levels decline in women, bone density also declines. Of course, there is some loss of bone seen with aging, and, as stated earlier, it tends to run in families. Then there are other factors that are not typically listed or discussed. One such factor is environmental toxins. Specifically, the heavy metals cadmium and lead. These are metals we are exposed to every day, often without knowing about the exposure. Both of these metals have been linked to causing osteoporosis.

Heavy metals and osteoporosis

Cadmium: Cadmium is a heavy metal that pollutes the air, waterways and soil. It is in food we eat that has been grown in contaminated soil, it is in the air we breathe thanks to industrial pollution, and it is in cigarette smoke. Cadmium has a high toxicity and stays in the body for 10 to 30 years after exposure. It has an affinity for the kidney and is often stored there, causing numerous kidney problems. Low-level cadmium exposure is associated with osteoporosis. Studies show that cadmium causes an increased excretion of calcium in the urine. The increased calcium loss due to cadmium exposure promotes bone demineralization and lower bone density.[1] A study done in Belgium in 1999 showed that post-menopausal women who had high urine cadmium levels had lower bone mineral density than women without high cadmium levels.[1] Other studies show that low-dose cadmium exposure interferes not only with calcium metabolism, but also with vitamin D and collagen metabolism.[2]

metals and undergoing heavy metal chelation can help decrease risk, but that involves visiting a physician who specializes in this area. If you think you have been exposed to heavy metals, there are some things you can do on your own.

Supplements and heavy metals:

♦ Zinc supplementation: An interesting study done in Japan showed that zinc supplementation stopped cadmium-induced bone loss.[7]

♦ NAC (N-acetylcysteine) supplementation: Has been shown to decrease lead toxicity.[8]

♦ Selenium and vitamin E help decrease metals.[9]

♦ Whey protein, milk thistle, and vitamin C all increase glutathione, which helps with metal toxicity.[9]

♦ Alpha lipoic acid helps decrease mercury.[9]

More in-depth environmental treatment is discussed later. If you already know you have osteopenia or osteoporosis, it is critical to seek treatment from your physician to stop the bone loss. Remember that if you are losing bone, you are probably releasing stored lead, which can cause hypertension and neurological and cognitive changes. The goal, of course, is to prevent bone loss by treating any known risk factors and removing any heavy metals that may be stored.

Polycystic Ovarian Syndrome (PCOS)

Polycystic ovarian syndrome is not really a disease, but is actually a number of symptoms that are grouped together and called a syndrome. Women who suffer from this condition typically display excess testosterone (called hyperandrogenism) and lack of ovulatory menstrual cycles. This often leads to infertility and can be the main reason a woman seeks treatment. Most women with PCOS have the classic symptoms of acne, obesity, hirsuitism (hair growth on the face, chest or abdomen) and irregular menstrual cycles. However, more and more often I'm seeing women with PCOS who don't fit the classic definition. Many PCOS women are of normal weight, have no excess hair growth, and may even have regular menses.

The most common symptoms are:

♦   Acne
♦   Weight gain and trouble losing weight
♦   Extra hair on the face and body
♦   Thinning hair on the scalp
♦   Infrequent or absent periods
♦   Lack of ovulation or infrequent ovulation which leads to fertility
    problems

Another characteristic that is used for diagnosis is the presence of numerous cysts inside the ovary. This is seen with a diagnostic pelvic ultrasound, and is described as looking like a string of pearls. But here again, not every woman with PCOS has this classic characteristic. To diagnose PCOS, first other causes of infrequent menses and excess androgens must be ruled out. The current diagnostic criteria is that at least two of the following three features must exist; oligo- or anovulation, clinical and/or laboratory signs of hyperandrogenism (excess testosterone), and polycystic ovaries seen by ultrasound (greater than 12 follicles 2-9 mm in size, or a volume greater than 10 ml).[1]

An important feature of polycystic ovarian syndrome is hormonal imbalance. This is not only testosterone imbalance but also insulin and blood sugar. PCOS patients often have elevated blood sugar and insulin levels, leading to metabolic disorders such as high cholesterol, insulin, and blood-sugar levels, and high blood pressure. How the hormones get out of balance in PCOS is poorly understood, but if left untreated will lead to infertility, diabetes and metabolic syndrome. What seems to be happening in PCOS is one hormone change triggers another, and then another. This causes a vicious circle of out-of-balance hormones.[2]

For example:

Normally, the ovaries make a tiny amount of male sex hormones (androgens). In PCOS, they start making slightly more androgens. This may cause a woman to stop ovulating, which will throw the menstrual cycle out of balance to the point that the cycle stops. The excess androgens also cause acne and extra facial and body hair. The body may then have a problem using insulin, called insulin resistance. When the body doesn't use insulin well, blood sugar levels go up. What comes first, the chicken or the egg? Some studies show that hyperandrogenism leads to high insulin levels in the blood, while other studies show that high insulin levels lead to high testosterone. The mechanism is difficult to understand, but what we do know is that there are correlations among high testosterone, high insulin and PCOS. Other hormones that are out of balance in women with PCOS are the follicle stimulating hormone (FSH) and the luteinizing hormone (LH). LH tends to be high and FSH low, causing a high LH-to-FSH ratio in 55% to 75% of women with PCOS. This imbalance will, of course, affect the menstrual cycle, ovulation and thus fertility.[3]

So how do hormones such as testosterone, FSH, LH and insulin get out of balance? This is where environmental toxins come into play. Remember that chemicals act like hormones in the body and can throw hormones out of balance.

Let's look at a few examples of chemicals linked to PCOS:

◆ Bisphenol-A
◆ Phthalates
◆ Heavy metals

Bisphenol-A(BPA) has the most research linking it to PCOS and insulin resistance. A study showed that mice injected with small amounts of bisphenol-A (doses matching their body weight) developed chronic high blood insulin levels and insulin resistance. [4] Although this is an animal study, it is interesting because the researchers compared BPA's effect on insulin to the hormone estradiol (E2). Low-dose estradiol had the same effect on insulin as did low-dose BPA, thus showing the estrogenic effects of BPA and its ability to alter hormones including insulin. Another study measured blood levels of BPA in women who were obese and had PCOS, and women who were not obese and had PCOS, and compared them to women without PCOS. The study found that women with PCOS had higher blood levels of BPA than women without PCOS and the size of the woman (obese or not obese) made no difference.[5] What is even more interesting about this study is that higher levels of BPA were also associated with high testosterone levels.

A 2005 study looked at blood levels of women with PCOS compared to controls and found the women with PCOS had more BPA in their blood than those without PCOS.[6] These studies are concerning, since BPA is present in so many sources, leading to widespread human exposure. BPA has been found in human fat tissue, blood, urine, breast milk and fetal blood. We are exposed to low doses every day from plastic food and beverage containers, metal food cans and dental sealants. Studies looking at low-dose exposure to BPA find a clear link to PCOS.

Phthalates are another chemical that affects women's hormones, the menstrual cycle, and ovulation. Phthalate is a general term for a class of chemicals found in plastics. A specific phthalate known as Di-2-ethylhexyl, or DEHP, is the most commonly used plasticizer for polyvinyl chloride products. PVC products include vinyl upholstery, shower curtains, tablecloths, raincoats, children's toys and more. The point is that we are exposed every day at some level. DEHP has been shown to alter hormone levels and cause anovulation. [7] DEHP has also been shown to suppress estradiol, which raises FSH, thus resulting in no LH surge and subsequent anovulation. This was one mechanism found to explain how phthalates cause PCOS.[8] Another mechanism is, again, through insulin resistance. Studies on men show a link between phthalate levels in the urine, insulin resistance and abdominal obesity. The effects were found to be due to phthalates' ability to alter hormones such as androgens. [9] This study shows that exposure to this common chemical can alter hormones, raise insulin levels, and increase obesity, which are factors in developing PCOS. This study clearly needs to be conducted on women to take the next obvious step and determine whether it's correlated it to PCOS.

Heavy metals such as mercury are known to cause disruption to a women's reproductive cycle. In a study looking at the affects of heavy metals on fertility, the body burden of heavy metals was measured and links made to PCOS.[11]   In the study of 501 women, 165 had signs of PCOS. They either had hyperandrogenism, hirsuitism, acne, polycystic ovaries on their ultrasounds or a combination of all of these. The study found elevated metals in women with PCOS, or signs of PCOS, and struggled with infertility.

Metal	**Condition**
Cadmium	Hirsuitism
Mercury	Hyperandrogenism
	Polycystic ovaries

We are exposed to these metals every day in small amounts through the air, our food, water and products. Cadmium is ingested with food that is grown in areas with contaminated water and soil. It also comes from different industries and is in fertilizer. Mercury has three forms. Organic mercury is from fish, seafood, pesticides and wood preservatives. Elemental mercury is from dental fillings, thermometers, fluorescent light bulbs and batteries. Inorganic mercury is in some skin care products and antiseptics.[10] Armed with this knowledge of what chemicals are linked to PCOS and how we are exposed to them, women can begin to take steps to avoid exposures and follow the treatment guidelines outlined in this book to remove chemicals from the body.

Summary

When a patient comes to see me for polycystic ovarian syndrome, I first determine if she is having issues with infertility and ask if getting pregnant is the goal. Often I am the one who makes the diagnosis of PCOS when patients come to see me for issues with fertility, acne, irregular menses, or problems losing weight. If the cause turns out to be PCOS, I determine if she has high blood sugar, insulin resistance or other metabolic factors that go with PCOS. Most conventional doctors would either put the patient on birth control pills to regulate her cycle or, if she was wanting to get pregnant, conventional doctors may use a drug called metformin to control the blood sugar and insulin problems in hopes that then she will ovulate and have normal cycles. Rarely do conventional doctors stop and ask, "Why does she have PCOS?" If they do ask "why," they assume the answer is because she is overweight, eats too much sugar and doesn't exercise. I look at the whole picture, including nutrition, exercise, lifestyle, menstrual cycle history and, of course, environmental toxins. I have found that incorporating naturopathic treatments for decreasing insulin resistance and testosterone helps with ovulation and the symptoms of PCOS, but the real treatment lies in the environmental approach. I take a history to determine what chemicals she may have been exposed to in her lifetime and offer testing for heavy metals, phthalates and BPA. Then I take her through an 8 week treatment plan to remove these chemicals and heavy metals from the body to rebalance the hormonal system and reverse PCOS.

Thyroid Disease

Thyroid disease seems to be an epidemic in this country. Over half of the women who come to see me in my practice have some sort of thyroid disorder ranging from hypothyroidism to hyperthyroidism. A large number of women with thyroid disease have the autoimmune forms called Hashimoto's and Graves' disease. Thyroid disease affects women eight times more often than men, and often occurs during pregnancy. The thyroid is a gland at the base of the neck right in front of the trachea. It produces two hormones that affect almost every organ in the body and regulates metabolism. The main hormone produced by the thyroid gland is thyroxine (T4) and a small amount of another hormone is also produced called triiodothyronine (T3). T3 is mostly made from the conversion of T4 in the blood or other tissues of the body. Hypothyroidism occurs when the thyroid gland does not produce enough thyroid hormone and metabolism slows down.

Signs of hypothyroidism include:

◆   Fatigue or weakness
◆   Weight gain
◆   Infrequent or absent menstrual periods
◆   Loss of sex drive
◆   Being cold or chilled easily
◆   Constipation
◆   Muscle aches
◆   Puffiness around the eyes
◆   Brittle nails
◆   Hair loss and dry skin

Hyperthyroidism means the gland is overactive and is producing too much thyroid hormone, causing the metabolism to increase.

Signs of hyperthyroidism include:

♦ Fatigue
♦ Weight loss
♦ Change in vision
♦ Nervousness
♦ Rapid heartbeat
♦ Increased sweating
♦ Being hot or overheating easily
♦ Menstrual spotting or frequent menses
♦ Frequent or loose bowel movements
♦ Tremor
♦ Anxiety and panic

Graves' disease is an autoimmune disorder where the body produces antibodies against the thyroid gland, causing it to produce too much thyroid hormone and thus leading to hyperthyroidism. Hashimoto's disease is an autoimmune condition as well, but it causes hypothyroidism.

What causes thyroid disease? It depends on what type of thyroid disease, but in general, there are common elements affecting the production of T4 and T3 from the thyroid gland as well as causing autoimmune thyroid disease.

Common risk factors include: [1,2,3]

♦ Pregnancy- 1 out of 50 women are diagnosed with hypothyroidism during pregnancy
♦ Estrogen therapy
♦ Stress
♦ Elevated cortisol

- Caloric restriction and anorexia
- Low selenium
- Low or high iodine intake
- Genetic
- Smoking
- Infections
- Systemic diseases
- Family history
- Medications such as lithium
- Exposure to radiation
- Environmental chemicals

Let's focus more on environmental chemicals. In my practice I have been successful at treating thyroid disease from an environmental medicine perspective. Some patients have been able to discontinue their medications by identifying and removing chemicals that triggered the thyroid disease. Even Graves' disease and Hashimoto's can be managed with cleansing and chelation. But first we have to know which toxins are linked to thyroid problems and know how chemicals interfere with the thyroid gland. Studies have shown that exposure in the womb or during lactation can affect the developing thyroid gland as well as exposure as a child or adult.[4]

The ways in which chemicals affect thyroid function include: [4, 14]

- Altering thyroid hormone metabolism
- Causing a direct toxic effect on the gland, changing function and regulation
- Producing thyroid antibodies (leading to autoimmune thyroid disorders)
- Interacting with thyroid-carrier proteins
- Blocking iodine uptake by the thyroid gland

Dr. Lyn Patrick published an amazing article in the 2009 issue of Alternative Medicine Review called "Thyroid disruption: mechanisms and clinical implications in human health." In it, she reviews the links to environmental chemicals and thyroid disease. The article is a must read for anyone wanting more detailed information on this condition.

The main chemicals that affect thyroid function are:

Polychlorinated Biphenols (PCBs) and dioxins. PCBs were once used in electrical transformers, capacitators, plasticizers and adhesives. Although many are no longer used in the U.S., they still persist in the environment. Eating fish from contaminated waters and farm raised fish is a means of exposure to PCBs, and so are dairy and meat products. Dioxin is formed as a byproduct of industrial processes involving chlorine such as waste incineration, chemical and pesticide manufacturing and paper bleaching. Dioxin was the primary toxic component of Agent Orange. The main way we are currently exposed to dioxin is through our food. It is a contaminant in meat, dairy and fish. PCBs and dioxins induce thyroid hormone metabolism through an enzyme called UDP-glucuronyl transferase. This simply means they alter liver function of the enzyme that metabolizes thyroid hormone. They also directly attack the thyroid gland and thyroid hormone carrier proteins.[5] There are numerous studies linking PCBs and dioxins to thyroid dysfunction.[6,7]

Pesticides have also been linked to thyroid disease in numerous studies. We are exposed to pesticides every day, whether we chose to be or not. They contaminate our air, water, food, soil, playground equipment, personal care products and more. There are numerous studies that link pesticides to thyroid dysfunction.

Maneb and mancozeb are pesticides sprayed on fruits such as bananas and have been found to alter the thyroid stimulating hormone (TSH), inhibit the thyroid peroxidase enzyme, and cause thyroid nodules.[8] A recent study of women married to men who sprayed pesticides on agriculture for a living had increased rates of thyroid disease. The study was published in January 8, 2010 online issue of the *American Journal of Epidemiology*. It looked at 16,500 women living in Iowa and North Carolina who were married to men using pesticides at work in the 1990s. Twelve-and-a-half percent of the women developed thyroid disease. This is a 1.2- to 1.4-fold increase from the general female population. It is interesting to note that these women didn't actually use the pesticides themselves, but were exposed secondhand through their husbands.

Pentachlorophenol (PCP) is a chemical used in industry. We are exposed without even knowing it exists. It is used as a wood preservative and produces toxic byproducts that contaminate our air, food and water. It too is linked to alteration of thyroid hormones and the formation of a goiter.[9] A goiter is an enlargement of the thyroid gland. It is not cancer, but typically is a signal that something is wrong with the gland.

Bisphenol-A (BPA) is another common chemical that we are exposed to every day through the lining of metal food cans, dental sealants and plastic bottles. It too is linked to thyroid disorders. Even at low doses consistent with what the average person would be exposed to; there are links to changes in thyroid hormones.[10]

Heavy metals are found to affect the thyroid as well. One of the main heavy metals studied is cadmium. Cadmium is a component of cigarette smoke and a product of industry. It is in the air, soil and water of most cities. We are exposed through cigarette smoke, food grown in contaminated soil, air pollution and water contamination. There are numerous studies linking thyroid disease to cadmium exposure. In one study, 636 children in Germany had their blood tested for thyroid hormones and correlated abnormalities to urine and blood levels of heavy metals. It was determined that children with alterations in thyroid hormones had high levels of cadmium in their blood.[11]

Mercury is also linked to thyroid disease in women and children. Methylmercury, which is found in fish, is linked to alterations in thyroid hormones via the mechanism of depleting selenium. Selenium is a mineral that is essential for proper thyroid function.[12]

Lead is another heavy metal that we are exposed to on a daily basis through our food, air and water. It too is linked to thyroid disorders in many studies. One study of note shows how sensitive a woman's hormonal system is compared to men's. Women's hormones appear to be more interconnected than men's hormones. For example, many women develop thyroid disease during pregnancy due to increases in estrogen and progesterone. One study compared men's and women's blood levels of lead and mercury to alterations in thyroid hormones and found that women were more affected by the heavy metals.[13]

Perchlorate. A recently published study showed a link between the chemical perchlorate and infant thyroid disorders. Perchlorate is used to make rocket fuel and explosives including fireworks. It is a contaminant in drinking water, breast milk and infant formula. A high urinary level of perchlorate was linked to high thyroid stimulating hormone (TSH) levels, which correlate with hypothyroidism. The thyroid disorders were only in infants with low iodine levels. Perchlorate and other chemicals are known to block iodine uptake by the thyroid gland, thus spelling out a mechanism of action for high TSH levels.[14] Perchlorate is also known to cause thyroid dysfunction in adults.

Perfluorooctanoic Acid (PFOA) is found in stain- and water-resistant coatings for carpet, furniture, fast-food containers, paints, and foams. These chemicals build up in our adipose tissue, or fat, and alter thyroid function. The National Health and Nutrition Examination Survey (NHANS) looked at 3,973 adults and measured PFOA levels. It determined high concentrations of PFOAs are linked to thyroid disease.[15]

Summary

When a patient comes to see me for treatment or management of a thyroid disorder I always ask, "Why?" Not why did they come to see me, but why do they have a thyroid problem? I feel too many doctors simply treat the symptoms of hypo or hyper-thyroidism and never ask why their patients' thyroids are not functioning properly. Few doctors take the time to try to find the cause or treat the cause. If a patient with hypothyroidism comes to see me, I tell them it is possible to get off the thyroid hormone. Some don't believe me. They had been told they would need it the rest of their lives. If a patient has hyperthyroidism, he or she is often told it's necessary to radiate and kill the thyroid or have it removed, thus making the patient hypothyroid, making it crucial to take thyroid hormone the rest of his or her life. The naturopathic medical students I teach often ask my opinion as to how I treat thyroid disease. I know from teaching for so long that what they are asking me is what type of thyroid hormone I would prescribe. They want to know if I'd prescribe what is considered synthetic thyroid verses what is considered natural thyroid. They are dumbfounded when I answer, "How do I treat thyroid? I treat the cause." They usually don't quite get what I am saying and ask point blank what hormone I use. This is when I launch into discussing the causes of thyroid disease and how to treat it. The most common cause I see is environmental chemicals.

I always take an environmental history on a patient, start a gentle cleanse, maybe offer some testing for toxins, maybe not, and always get good results. Of course, I first rule out the other causes that are mentioned above.

The most success I have is with hypothyroidism and hyperthyroidism. I do have success using this approach with Graves' disease and Hashimotos' disease, although they are much more challenging given the autoimmune component.

Chapter III Summary

This chapter was meant to provide you with scientific evidence linking common women's health conditions to chemicals in the environment. An entire book could be written about each condition so I tried to keep it simple. Other health conditions affecting women, men and children are also linked to chemicals in the environment. Every day the body of evidence grows, and it is time we ask that these chemicals stay out of our food, air, water and products. That calls for tighter regulation or for industries to stop using them altogether and look for safer, healthier alternatives.

Chapter IV
What's in your body?
(Testing)

This chapter is meant to be a guide to help you understand what type of testing needs to be considered. In the resource section I list the labs I use, but there are many labs across the country that run environmental tests looking for heavy metals, solvents, pesticides and other chemicals. Some of the tests are covered by insurance carriers, and others are not. If I take a really good history to determine what someone's exposures have been and correlate that to symptoms or current health conditions, I am often able to head straight to treatment. However, some people want to know the levels of chemicals in their body, so testing should be offered. Also, by testing before and after treatment you are able to objectively track the amount of chemicals that are removed from the body versus basing improvement on symptoms alone.

If heavy metal toxicity is suspected, it is important to test for these metals in the body because the treatment is more complex than simple detoxification. Heavy metal testing can be cheap and easy, so, at a minimum, run that test. Also, if you recall from reading about the health conditions, some people are genetically set up to have trouble breaking down or clearing toxins through the liver. Those genetic changes are determined by a blood test that I also like to run on people.

Where to begin with testing?

Initially, a general blood panel is required to determine if the immune system is functioning properly and to establish that the organs of elimination, such as the kidney and liver, are working well. These tests can be ordered by any doctor and are covered by insurance. They include a complete blood count, complete metabolic panel, lipid panel, thyroid panel, urine creatine level and vitamin D test.

The next test I like to run gives great information about the liver's ability to break down medications, herbs, chemicals and your own body's hormones. This is a test for genetic alterations in the enzymes that control liver phase-one and phase-two detoxification pathways. These genetic changes are called single nucleotide polymorphisms, or SNPs.

Phase-one liver cytochrome P450 enzymes:

- CYP1A1
- CYP1A2
- CYP1B1
- CYP2A6
- CYP2C9
- CYP2C19
- CYP2D6
- CYP2E1
- CYP3A4

Liver phase-two conjugation reactions:

- COMT
- NAT1
- NAT2
- GSTM1
- GSTP1
- SOD

Each of these enzyme pathways in the liver is responsible for metabolizing medications, herbs, hormones, and chemicals. Labs that offer this test will provide a detailed list of what is broken down by each pathway that has a single nucleotide polymorphism (SNP). This will allow for an individualized treatment plan supporting the pathway that is having trouble breaking down chemicals.

Heavy metal testing

There are basically two reliable methods of testing for levels of heavy metals in the body: blood and urine. Heavy metals are present in small amounts in the air, water, food and products. They are fat-loving compounds and may stay stored in the body for decades. Performing a heavy metal test that accurately reflects what has built up in the body from years of exposure would mean running a blood or urine test. Some might think a hair analysis is a good place to start, since it is cheap and easy to perform. A hair analysis does not offer an accurate picture of heavy metals that are stored in the body's tissue. It often shows inaccurate results due to contamination from air pollution, chemicals in the water to which the hair is exposed during showering, and chemicals in various hair products. It only gives a snapshot of recent exposure of metals still circulating in the blood and does not give an accurate picture of what is stored in the body.[1,2]

The Agency for Toxic Substances and Disease Registry (ATSDR) explored the reliability and validity of hair analysis and states: "Before hair analysis can be considered a valid tool for any particular substance, research is needed to establish better reference ranges, gain a better understanding of hair biology and pharmacokinetics, further explore possible dose-response relationships, establish whether and when hair may serve as a better measure or predictor of disease than other biological samples (e.g., blood or urine), and learn more about organic compounds in hair."

Blood measurement of heavy metals can show what is present in the body at the time the blood is drawn.[3] Blood testing a good measurement of current exposure but not of what is stored in the body, referred to as body burden. Most commercial labs offering blood heavy metal testing have reference ranges set primarily for high dose, acute heavy metal poisoning.[4] The reference ranges are often set too high to detect low dose, chronic heavy metal exposure.

Urine heavy metal testing typically includes both a "pre-challenge", also called "un-provoked", and a "post-challenge" or "provoked" urine collection. A pre-challenge test is a random urine collection and is a good measurement of chronic metal exposure. According to the ATSDR, "urine tests provide the best estimates of the current body burden of chronic mercury poisoning. Elemental and inorganic mercury are mainly excreted in the urine". A pre-challenge, unprovoked, urine test shows what metals are currently circulating in the body and being excreted by the kidney. It is important to make sure kidney function is intact prior to testing. If levels are high on an unprovoked test it means there is a current exposure to heavy metals. Some labs are using outdated reference ranges giving the appearance of a normal urine metal test. The Centers for Disease Control has set new US references ranges for metals in the urine. These ranges are tighter than most commercial labs. *http://www. cdc.gov/exposurereport*

After completing an unprovoked or pre-challenge urine test to determine what the patient is currently being exposed to, a provoked or post-challenge urine heavy metal test should be run to determine past or chronic exposure to heavy metals. A provoked urine test involves giving a body weight dose of heavy metal chelator to the patient to pull metals from storage sites. Prior to administering this test the physician must run a complete blood count and comprehensive metabolic panel to ensure the liver and kidneys are functioning properly. After giving the dose of chelator the urine is collected for 6 hours and sent to the lab. A chelator binds minerals from the body as well as metals. Therefore it is necessary to replace minerals after a post-challenge test.

The downside to provocative heavy metal testing is that there are no set reference ranges. Labs that offer heavy metal testing set reference ranges for unprovoked urine testing and not provoked. So if a patient's test comes back with elevated levels of heavy metals I often ask, elevated in relation to what? Typically I will compare each patient's unprovoked urine test to their provoked urine test to determine if more heavy metals are in the body then what a random urine collection showed. Many physicians feel that a provoked urine test gives an estimate of body burden of metals. However, there is no way to know where the increase in heavy metal excretion is coming from on a provoked test. For example if lead shows up elevated on a provoked urine test is it merely circulating lead being pulled through the kidney, is it coming from the bone, extracellular spaces, or other sites. No matter where it is coming from it typically represents past or chronic exposure.

There are three forms of chelating agents typically used to perform this test. DMSA (dimercaptosuccinic acid), DMPS (2,3-dimercapto-1-propanesulfonic acid), and EDTA (ethylenediaminetetraacetic acid). DMSA is administered orally and the other two intravenously. All should be administered by a doctor trained in environmental medicine.[5]

Testing for other chemicals

Numerous labs offer blood and urine tests for chemicals such as solvents, pesticides, formaldehyde (as formic acid in the urine), parabens, phthalates, and more. Some labs test for pesticides and solvents and offer different panels, so taking a thorough history is important in order to choose a panel with the solvents or pesticides most likely to be in the body. Phthalates can be tested for in the urine by several labs (see resource section). There is no provocative or challenge test for these chemicals, so both blood and urine will give circulating levels. I often try to get the body to release stored chemicals before running a urine or blood test. I do this by having the patient fast for 24 hours and/or go into a hot sauna before the test. Both caloric restriction and sauna therapy have shown to increase blood and urine levels respectively. This will be discussed in depth in the chapter on treatment.

There are many options for testing what chemicals are stored or circulating in the body. It is not necessary to know the levels prior to performing treatment, but it gives an objective indication (beyond symptom improvement) that the treatment is working and toxins are being removed from the body.

CHAPTER V
THE WORLD IS SUCH A BIG PLACE!
WHAT'S A GIRL TO DO?
(AVOIDANCE)

It is clear by now that we are all exposed to chemicals on some level every day of our lives. It is also clear that these chemicals are linked to serious health conditions. Now it is time to make clear that by avoiding these chemicals in the first place, we may be able to prevent health conditions that affect thousands of women each year. So where does one begin? This chapter is broken down into sections on how to avoid exposures in the food, water, air and common products we all use almost every day. I will focus on the home, since that is where we spend most of our time, but keep in mind that the work environment is another place where we breathe the air, drink the water and are exposed to carpet, cleaning products, perfume and personal grooming products. What you learn here should be shared with everyone you know, with the goal of helping everyone to live in a chemical free world.

Food

Here are seven simple tips to avoid chemicals in your food.

1.   Eat only organic fruits and vegetables to avoid pesticide
     residue. If you must eat non-organic fruits and vegetables,
     refer to the Environmental Working Group's list of foods high
     and low in pesticide residue www.ewg.org

     The 12 most toxic fruits and vegetables:

     ♦   Peaches
     ♦   Apples
     ♦   Bell peppers
     ♦   Celery
     ♦   Nectarines
     ♦   Strawberries
     ♦   Cherries
     ♦   Kale
     ♦   Lettuce
     ♦   Grapes (imported)
     ♦   Carrots
     ♦   Pears

     The 12 least toxic fruits and vegetables:

     ♦   Onions
     ♦   Avocados
     ♦   Sweet corn
     ♦   Pineapples
     ♦   Mangos
     ♦   Asparagus
     ♦   Sweet peas
     ♦   Kiwi
     ♦   Cabbage

♦ Eggplant
♦ Papaya
♦ Watermelon

2. Eat only wild fish, not farmed fish, and eat wild fish low in mercury. The following information is from the Centers for Disease Control and Environmental Working Group.

Fish low in mercury:

♦ Wild salmon
♦ Catfish (highly farm raised fish)
♦ Clams
♦ King crab
♦ Flounder
♦ Oysters
♦ Sole
♦ Sardines
♦ Scallops
♦ Shrimp
♦ Tilapia (highly farm raised fish)

Fish with moderate amounts of mercury:

♦ Grouper
♦ Halibut
♦ Pollock
♦ Sablefish
♦ Sea trout
♦ Cod
♦ Crab, Dungeness and blue
♦ Haddock
♦ Herring
♦ Mahi mahi
♦ Ocean perch

- Tuna, canned, light
- Whitefish

Fish high in mercury:

- King mackerel
- Shark
- Swordfish
- Tilefish
- Bluefish
- Lobster
- Marlin
- Orange roughy
- Red snapper
- Bass (saltwater)
- Trout (freshwater)
- Tuna (fresh)
- Tuna, canned, white albacore

3. Buy fresh food when possible, and avoid food stored in plastic or food in cans lined with plastic. Two companies confirmed to have cans free of Bisphenol-A are Eden and Vital Choice. A few of the Trader Joe's canned foods are free of BPA but not all.

4. Eat only organic meat and dairy products to avoid added hormones, pesticides and PCBs.

5. Eat meat and fish cooked at low temperatures and avoid grilled or charbroiled meat and fish. Remember that high temperature cooking creates polyaromatic hydrocarbons, (PAHs).

6. Drink water and other beverages from glass containers or stainless steel bottles. Avoid plastic beverage bottles. If you must drink out of plastic, look for bottles that state they are

free of Bisphenol-A. Also, flip the bottle over and look at the number on the bottom. Avoid plastic bottles with the numbers: **#1, #3, #6, #7**

7. Try to avoid the use of plastic food storage containers or plastic cling wrap on your food. Instead, use glass storage containers, and if you need to wrap your food, use paper.

Water

You would think that living in a developed country such as the United States, one wouldn't have to worry about the water quality. That thought is only partially true. The water in the U.S. is treated with disinfectants, so it is free of waterborne diseases common in undeveloped countries. However, your water is not as clean and pure as you might think.

Some common sources of water contamination include:

Agriculture   Pesticides, herbicides, defoliants

Industrial   Formaldehyde, phenols, detergents, phthalates, pesticides, PCBs

Purification   Chlorination, ozone

Conduits/pipes   Lead, copper, PVC.

Some drinking water contains pharmaceutical medications, pesticides, solvents, heavy metals, and byproducts from the disinfectant process. These chemicals are discussed in detail in Chapter Two. You can see which contaminants are in your local drinking water by searching the Environmental Working Group database. *www.ewg.org*

I recommend filtering the water you drink and use for cooking and bathing. Water filtration can remove most chemicals and impurities. First, you should have your water at home tested for chemical contaminants so you know what you need to filter out. Your local city water department offers testing, as do some specialty labs and companies. Doctors Data Lab in Illinois offers inexpensive water testing for heavy metals. National Testing Laboratories in Ohio offers a more in-depth water analysis called Watercheck. The Center for Environmental Quality at Wilkes University has free informational documents available on water quality issues and also offers testing of drinking water. Each laboratory will have reference ranges for the acceptable amounts of the chemicals that may be in your water. I recommend using the guidelines set forth by the Environmental Protection Agency (EPA) and the Centers for Disease Control (CDC).

Once you know what is in your water, you need to filter it out. If you discover very high levels of a particular chemical, I also suggest you notify your local water department and the local news station so others can be alerted to the possible dangers lurking in the water. Once the water has been tested and you know what chemicals are in the water, purchase a filtration system designed to remove the chemicals of concern. Home water treatment systems are of two basic types, either point-of-use or point-of-entry.

Point-of-use devices treat water within the home, such as at the kitchen sink or at the showerhead. If the chemical is only a concern for when you are cooking, bathing or drinking the water in the kitchen, then a point-of-use system is fine.

A point-of-entry or *whole house* system treats all the water coming into the house from the city line. This is recommended for chemicals such as radon and volatile organic compounds (VOC). This is why you first need to know what chemicals are in your water.

What type of filter should you buy?

There are several different types of filtration devices on the market, and it can be confusing to the consumer as to which one is the best. Again, it depends on what you want to filter and where in the house you want to filter the water. A nonprofit organization called NSF International does a good job of rating the various types of filtration systems available. They also certify units according to strict standards and guidelines. Go to *www.nsf.org* for a list of certified filtration systems.

Here are a few examples of different filtration systems available for the home:

♦ Activated charcoal/carbon
♦ Reverse osmosis
♦ Aeration
♦ Distillation
♦ Ion exchange
♦ Ultraviolet light

Activated charcoal/carbon is the most common type of filter that people buy. This is the pour-through container where water is passed over the filter and collects into a plastic pitcher. They are effective for removing radon, organic chemicals, chlorine, odors, some VOCs and pesticides, lead, and trihalomethanes. These units can be connected to the kitchen sink, showerhead, point-of-entry, and the manual-fill pitchers. The filter must be changed every two to three months or bacteria will grow. Point-of-entry use is the most effective location for charcoal/carbon filters.

Reverse osmosis (RO) is effective for removing heavy metals, asbestos, some pesticides, VOCs, and trihalomethanes. Most RO systems are point-of-use and placed under the kitchen sink. They typically come with the filter membrane plus a pre- and post-filter.

These need to be changed every six months to avoid the growth of bacteria. The downside of RO systems is the amount of wastewater created during the filtration process. As the water is being treated, it is collected in a storage container and the impurities and chemicals are washed away in a stream of wastewater. A RO unit may take almost three hours to produce one gallon of treated water from several gallons of contaminated water. So, yes, a lot of water is wasted in this process.

Aeration is a point-of-entry system that can remove very high levels of radon and VOCs, so it is not necessary for the average contaminants in water. Air is introduced into the water to volatize these chemicals, which are then vented and released into the air. This, of course, becomes a source of air pollution. There are three types of aeration devices: a packed tower, bubble aerator and spray aerator. These need to be professionally installed and are expensive to maintain.

Distillation is one of the oldest methods of water treatments. These are point-of-use systems effective for removing arsenic, some pesticides, and organic chemicals including heavy metals. The process is energy intensive, as the water is heated into steam and then cooled back to water, leaving any chemicals behind. There are two types, air-cooled and water-cooled. Air-cooled produces one gallon of distilled water from one gallon of tap water. Water-cooled makes one gallon of distilled water from 5 to 15 gallons of tap water. This method is not good for VOCs, trihalomethanes and some pesticides.

Ion exchange replaces chemicals with ions, such as sodium or chloride. The most common type of ion exchange is a water softener system. The other type is called an "anion exchange device". These can remove some heavy metals, but they mostly remove hard minerals and salts. They can leave behind high levels of sodium in the water.

Ultraviolet light systems radiate the water to remove chemicals, micro-organisms, spores and viruses. They don't remove heavy metals, VOCs, or pesticides. They are energy intensive, and the bulbs can be expensive.

Is bottled water a safe option?

Many people use bottled water at home for their drinking and cooking water. Obviously it can't be used for showering or bathing. The Food and Drug Administration (FDA) is the organization that regulates the bottled water industry, and the FDA has established standards in regards to the quality of bottled water. The standards are similar to the acceptable levels set by the EPA. However, the FDA does not always check the bottled water industry to see if they are following the guidelines. The other concern regarding bottled water is the use of plastics. This has already been discussed in length in Chapters Two and Three. Hard and soft bottled water has chemicals in it that are known hormone disruptors in women. I advise against the use of any plastic beverage bottle. Instead, get your home water tested and consult a professional on which home water filtration system is best for you. Then put your filtered water into a stainless steel bottle or glass bottle for use when you are away from the house.

Air

Cleaning up the air is easier and less expensive than cleaning up your drinking water. It starts with treating the cause of the poor air quality. You may not think you have control over outdoor air quality, but you actually have more control than you might think. You can get involved in your local city government and push for tighter restrictions on emissions from cars, trucks, and public transportation. Since most outdoor air pollution is caused by industry and coal-burning power plants, you might consider electing public officials willing to take on these industries or get involved in environmental groups that address this cause. You can get involved in your neighborhood association or homeowners' association and restrict the use of toxic pesticides that are sprayed on lawns, at local parks and on golf courses. You can help set limits on when people in your city can burn fires in the fireplace. Some cities in California and Arizona have no-burn days depending on the air quality for that day.

Obviously it is easier to clean up your air at home since you are the one making decisions regarding what type of cleaning and grooming products, pesticides, and other chemicals you use in your home. Remember from Chapter Two that indoor air is more toxic than outdoor air. It is important to make healthy choices regarding furniture, paint, mattresses, building materials, carpeting and anything else that can emit harmful chemicals and create unhealthy indoor air quality. I will discuss alternatives to these products later in this chapter.

Common chemicals found in indoor air are: [1]

♦ Formaldehyde
♦ Toluene
♦ Xylene
♦ Benzene
♦ Phthalates
♦ Trichloroethane

Common sources of these chemicals are: [1]

♦ Carpet
♦ Cleaning products
♦ Vinyl flooring
♦ Dry-cleaning fluids on clothes
♦ Floor polish
♦ Carpet shampoo

♦ Cigarettes
♦ Air fresheners
♦ Mattresses
♦ Furniture

There are simple tests and devices that can alert you to harmful chemicals in the air. I recommend that every home should have a carbon monoxide (CO) detector and get checked for Radon. You can order an inexpensive radon check kit at *www.radon.com*. You should not use unvented heaters in your home. This includes an unvented wood-burning fireplace and an unvented natural gas fireplace. Avoid an unvented natural gas space heater and all unvented natural gas appliances. Keep your air conditioning and heating ducts and vents clean and have regular maintenance checks on these units.

The simplest thing you can do at home to improve your indoor air quality is use an air filter in the bedroom and the living room. Different airborne chemicals are of different particle sizes, meaning some are really small and some are really big. Particles 10 microns or less in size can enter our respiratory tracts, noses, mouths and lungs. This size particle can also enter our blood and lymph systems. Most household chemical contaminants such as tobacco smoke, pesticides, cooking smoke, dust and mold are 5 micros or less and can easily cause health problems. It is important to choose an air filter that removes small particles from the air. There are professionally installed whole house air filters and buy-at-the-store room air filters. Both *www.consumerreports.org* and *www.air-purifier-power.com* rate room air filters. A widely accepted voluntary program that certifies air filters is the Association of Home Appliance Manufactures.

There are different types of household room air filters, including:

♦ HEPA filters
♦ ULPA filters
♦ Electrostatic filters
♦ Ionization
♦ Ozone
♦ Carbon filters

HEPA stands for "high efficiency particulate filter." A fan draws air through a paper or fine mesh filter. It removes 99.97% of all airborne pollutants 0.3 microns or larger as long as the unit is kept cleaned and the filter is changed according to manufacturer specifications.

ULPA stands for "ultra-HEPA filter" and works the same way as a HEPA filter but is designed to trap 99.99% of airborne particles 0.3 microns or larger.

Electrostatic filters or precipitators have a synthetic membrane barrier that creates static electricity as the air flows over it. A positive charge is applied to air particles flowing past metal plates. The charged particles stick to the negatively charged plate just like clothes with static cling stick together. These create some ozone as a byproduct. This is called ground level ozone and can be harmful or irritating to the lungs. Consumer reports tested these filters in October 2003 and December 2007 and found that electrostatic filters were less effective than HEPA filters at removing pollutants.

Ionization is a method of room air filtration in which particles are drawn in and ionized, or given a negative charge. These newly negatively charged particles are released back into the air and fall onto furniture, walls and floors, which are positively charged. This does create dust in the home which can be stirred back up with movement or a draft.

Ozone generators draw air over a high voltage plate. Oxygen molecules pass through the electric discharge and are ionized, combining with oxygen to form ozone. The ozone theoretically kills organisms in the air and on surfaces. These are the least efficient at removing harmful particulates and the safety of ground level ozone has been questioned.

Carbon filters absorb volatile organic chemicals by passing air through a large carbon filter. A large surface area and contact time is required, and it is not as efficient when it comes to removing small particles as a HEPA system is.

It is also important to filter the air you breathe while traveling in the car and on an airplane. Most new cars come equipped with HEPA air filters in the dashboard, but you must remember to change them often. Personal air filters that can be worn around your neck for air travel are available at various stores and Internet sites. You also can get a filter for your car that plugs into the lighter and provides additional filtration while driving.

Plants are nature's air filters. Not only do they brighten a room and add decoration, but they can clean your air, too.

When choosing plants, consider: [2]

♦ Boston Ferns (the number-one air purifier)
♦ Areca palms
♦ Lady palms
♦ Bamboo Palm (good for removing solvents)
♦ Rubber plants (excellent for formaldehyde)
♦ English Ivy
♦ Dwarf date palms (good for removing xylene)
♦ Peace lilies
♦ Golden Pothos
♦ Dracaena Janet Craig

Home

By now you are aware of the dangers of conventional products used at home or on the body. They contain chemicals, or toxins, that affect your health. In the previous chapters I described how you are exposed to these chemicals and what health conditions are linked to their exposure. In the next chapter, I describe treatments you can do to remove these toxins from your body and improve your health. But avoidance is the most important thing you can do to protect yourself. This is the section where I will list alternatives to the standard products used at home. Making informed choices at the store will send a clear message to companies that we don't want these harmful chemicals in our products. This information is gathered from numerous sources.[1,2,3,4,5] Most safe products are now commercially available at a store near you. In the section on resources, I list where you can buy the harder-to-find items.

Products

Cleaning products contain harmful chemicals such as surfactants, solvents, volatile organic compounds, synthetic dyes and fragrances, brighteners, anti-microbial agents and inert ingredients. The chemical names are nothing we haven't already heard by now. Instead of buying the standard products, which are loaded with harmful chemicals, try making your own cleaning products and detergents. A great resource is a book by Patricia Thomas called *What's in this stuff?* Here are some examples from the Women's Health & Environmental Network (WHEN).

Air Freshener
Leave an open bowl of lavender or rosemary out on the shelf. This will remove odors. Change frequently.

All Purpose Cleaner
Mix 1/2 cup vinegar and 1/2 cup water in a spray bottle. This is a great all purpose cleaner and window cleaner.

Disinfectant Cleaner
Mix 1/2 cup borax and 1 gallon of hot water. You can put this in a spray bottle or use in a bucket with a sponge or mop depending on what you need to clean.

Drain Cleaner
Always use a drain basket and hair catcher in the shower and kitchen to prevent hair from going down the drain. Clear clogs with 1/4 cup of baking soda followed by 1/2 cup of white vinegar, then flush with hot water. Don't forget you can use a plunger and metal drain snake to remove clogs.

Furniture Polish
Try 3 parts olive oil and 1 part vinegar with a little lemon juice to scent the oil.

Floor Cleaners
1 cup vinegar or borax in 1 gallon of warm water works for linoleum, tile, brick or stone. Warm/hot water with a few drops of olive oil for wood floors.

Oven cleaners
Use baking soda and hot water to make a paste and use this to scour the inside of ovens. Steel wool and pumice stone will remove black spots.

Toilet Cleaners
Borax, vinegar and baking soda with water are all good options—plus a little elbow grease. A pumice stone is great to remove stains as well.

Listed below is a sampling of non-toxic commercial products that are available at a store near you. More companies than listed here do exist and can be found at *www.organicconsumers.org* and *www. thegreenguide.com*.

Laundry detergents:

- Seventh Generation
- Life Tree
- Sun and Earth
- Ecover
- BioKleen
- Oxi-Clean
- Bio Pac
- Nature Clean
- Earthrite

Dishwashing detergents:

- Seventh Generation
- Citra Solv
- Ecover
- Nature Clean

Glass cleaners and all-purpose cleaners:

- Dr. Bronners
- Seventh Generation
- BioKleen
- Green Clean
- Bon Ami

Air fresheners:

♦ Earth Friendly Uni-Fresh
♦ Air Sense Natural Air

Toilet cleaner:

♦ Ecover
♦ Green Clean
♦ Bon Ami

Wood polish:

♦ Citra-wood
♦ Earthrite furniture polish
♦ Seventh Generation

Beauty and cosmetic products

This category is harder to simply provide a list of non-toxic products for, due to the misleading labeling on many products. The words "natural" or "organic" don't necessarily mean a product is free of harmful chemicals. You have to educate yourself on what the chemical name means and READ THE LABEL. A great resource is a book by Paula Begoun called *Don't Go to the Cosmetics Counter Without Me.*

Some chemicals you want to avoid in products include:

♦ Sodium or Ammonium Lauryl or Laureth Sulphate
♦ Sodium Methyl Cocoyl Taurate
♦ Sodium Lauroyl or Cocoyl Sarcosinate
♦ Cocomidopropyl Betaine
♦ TEA compounds
♦ DEA compounds

- PEG (Polyethylene Glycol) compounds
- Quarternium -7,15,31,60 etc.
- Lauryl or Cocoyl Sarcosine
- Disodium Oleamide or Dioctyl Sulfosuccinate
- Propylene Glycol
- Ethylene/Diethylene Glycol
- PEG compounds (e.g. Polyethylene Glycol)
- Cetyl Alcohol (organic co-emulsifier)
- Sodium Hydroxide (pH adjuster)
- Sorbic Acid (organic compound)
- Tocopherol Acetate (vitamin E Derivative)
- Methyl Paraben
- Propyl Paraben
- Imidazolidinyl Urea (organic compound)
- Fragrance
- FD and C Yellow No. 5, D7C Red No. 33

The Organic Consumers Association looks at which companies are making false claims in regards to the non-toxic nature of their products. For example, at *www.organicconsumers.org/bodycare*, they outline some companies and products who claim to be organic or natural when in reality they contain harmful chemicals.

Here is a sample of companies who make "false claims", according to Organic Consumers Association:

- Avalon "Organics"
- Desert Essence "Organics"
- Earth's Best "Organic"
- Eminence "Organic" (except a few with a USDA seal)
- Giovanni "Organic"
- Goodstuff "Organics"
- Head "Organics"
- Jason "Pure, Natural & Organic"
- Kiss My Face "ObsessivelyOrganic"

◆   Nature's Gate "Organics"
◆   Physicians Formula "Organic" Wear
◆   Stella McCartney "100% Organic"

Source: Organic Consumers Association 6771 South Silver Hill Drive, Finland, MN 55603

The Organic Consumers Association recommends sticking with USDA-certified beauty products, such as:

◆   Alteya Organics
◆   Aubrey Organics
◆   Baby Bear Shop
◆   Badger
◆   Brittanie's Thyme
◆   Bubble and Bee Organic
◆   Dr. Bronner's Magic Soaps
◆   Earth Mama Angel Baby
◆   Indian Meadow Herbals
◆   Intelligent Nutrients
◆   Kimberly Parry Organics
◆   Little Angel
◆   Mercola
◆   Miessence Certified Organics
◆   Nature's Paradise
◆   OGmama and OGbaby
◆   Organicare
◆   Organic Essence
◆   Origins Organics
◆   Purely Shea
◆   Rose Tattoo Aftercare
◆   SoCal Cleanse
◆   Sensibility Soaps/Nourish
◆   Terressentials
◆   Trillium Organics
◆   Vermont Soap

Source: Organic Consumers Association 6771 South Silver Hill Drive, Finland, MN 55603

The Environmental Working Group recently compiled a cosmetic safety database called Skin Deep. You can enter in the name of a cosmetic and find out if it contains harmful ingredients (*www. cosmeticdatabase.com*).

Another group that reviews cosmetics is www.safecosmetics.org. This group has a list of cosmetic companies that have signed an agreement to keep harmful chemicals out of cosmetic and beauty products. You can find the list of companies on their website under "Companies," and can search for responsible companies who signed the Compact for Safe Cosmetics.

Home and Building Products

Every building material, carpet, furniture and even mattresses can contain harmful chemicals. There are options available. Look under the resource section of this book to find alternatives for every need for your home.

Paints
Non-toxic paints would be formaldehyde-free, acetone-free, zero or low-volatile organic compound (VOC) paint with zero VOC pigments.

Flooring
Examples of non-toxic flooring available include: cork, natural linoleum, solid bamboo, Forest Stewardship Council (FSC)-certified wood, reclaimed wood, recycled terrazo tiles, rubber, natural wool rugs, natural fiber carpets, virtually zero-emitting carpet pads, recycled porcelain tiles and soy-based concrete stain.

Tile can be toxic, so look for safe options such as: recycled glass tile, recycled fused glass tile, recycled porcelain tile, recycled ceramic tile.

Countertops

Non-toxic counters include bamboo butcher block, recycled glass and concrete, and FSC PaperStone surfaces.

Cabinets

Look for cabinets made without formaldehyde and use non-toxic paints, finishes, and sealants.

Particleboard and sheets

Look for bamboo plywood, bamboo veneers, sorghum stalk plywood, formaldehyde-free particleboard and formaldehyde-free, medium-density fiberboard.

Carpet

Look for wool, biodegradable, formaldehyde-free and flame-retardant free.

Mattresses

No latex or synthetic fillers should be present, as well as no synthetic glues, dyes, or finishing spays used in any stage of production. They should be formaldehyde and flame retardant free.

Summary

Some of this information may be familiar to you, and some may be new. The information is meant to empower you to make healthy choices in regards to food, water and products, and to keep your air free of chemicals. The products listed that are deemed safe or unsafe come from several sources, which are referenced (the author has no personal interest in any cosmetic or cleaning product company).

Lists may seem overwhelming, so I made a simple summary of where to begin as you strive to avoid chemicals in your life.

Summary on avoiding toxins in your daily life:

- Buy only organic fruits and vegetables that are free of pesticide residues.
- Buy hormone and antibiotic free meats and dairy products.
- Buy fresh or frozen foods and avoid canned foods.
- Eat wild fish low in mercury, like wild Alaskan salmon, blue crab, flounder, haddock, Pollack, and trout.
- Do not store or heat food in plastic containers; use glass.
- Buy in bulk to decrease plastic packaging.
- Store food in glass jars when you get it home.
- Carry groceries in cloth bags and reuse them instead of using plastic bags.
- Drink water out of glass containers rather than plastic.
- Filter your own water.
- Use a home air filter.
- Consider a personal air filter for the car or travel.
- Use earth-friendly, simple detergent, cleaners and soaps.
- Try to rework your conception of what looks beautiful, and avoid herbicides and pesticides.
- Use natural pest control instead of insecticides.
- Replace vinyl mini blinds, shower curtains, and placemats with fabric.
- If you're building a home or remodeling, use earth-friendly, non-toxic materials.
- Use a non-toxic drycleaner, or air out dry-cleaning before bringing it into the home.
- Remove your shoes when you enter the home.
- Use natural, organic, non-bleached tampons without a plastic applicator.
- Avoid the use of fragrances, and remember that unscented is not fragrance free.
- Use only non-toxic cosmetics, lotions, shampoos, deodorant and other products.

CHAPTER VI
HOW DO YOU GET THIS STUFF OUT?
(TREATMENT)

Whenever I give a talk about environmental toxins and health to physicians, students, or the public, at some point I stop and say: even though we are bombarded every day with chemicals that make us ill, we can't become paranoid about the environment. It can be overwhelming, and some may think they can't breathe the air, eat food, drink water, drive a car, or go out in public. You may feel like hiding indoors or living in a bubble. But you can't do that. Instead, what you can do is take yourself through a detoxification plan and then practice the chapter on avoidance to minimize exposure to toxins. Since it is impossible to completely avoid toxins, you can cleanse once or twice a year to prevent any health problems. If you have a health condition you think is linked to toxins, you can detoxify or cleanse to improve or reverse the problem. The words "detox," "detoxify," "detoxification" and "cleanse" are used interchangeably throughout this chapter.

The basic principle behind detoxification is to remove the toxins stored in your body. This is done by releasing chemicals from fat tissue, organs and extracellular spaces that have been stored for years. Once they are released, they will reenter the blood stream and be metabolized through the liver. This is where it is critical to support liver phase-one and phase-two detoxification pathways.

The liver is where toxins are broken down in order to be eliminated. Next, the organs of elimination need to be supported to get the toxic byproducts produced from the liver out of the body.

The organs of elimination include:

♦ Kidneys
♦ Bowels
♦ Skin
♦ Lungs

We eliminate through urination, moving our bowels, sweating and breathing. If these organs don't function properly, then toxins get re-circulated back into the body and are stored. For example, if someone is constipated or doesn't ever sweat, then he or she is not eliminating toxins.

The principles of detoxification are simple, and the mechanism of supporting the liver and organs of elimination is well proven. For example, there are many mechanisms that can be pointed to in regards to how a particular nutrient or plant affects a particular pathway in the liver. Critics of the environmental medicine approach to treating disease point to a lack of published results of full treatment protocols around detoxification and cleansing that show a resolution of disease. However, there is research in this area on each piece of the whole plan, and I include it throughout this chapter. I have been utilizing this treatment approach with patients for a decade and have seen great results.

Note: Prior to beginning any type of treatment plan you must consult with your physician to determine if you have any health problems that would prevent you from following this plan. Also, remember that over-the-counter vitamins, minerals, herbs and other supplements can interact with prescription medications and with each other so consult a professional.

Mobilization

The release of stored chemicals from fat tissue and organs is quite involved. Some of these chemicals have been stored for years and are tightly bound to tissues. The first part of detoxification involves getting the stored toxins to be released back into the blood stream.

Methods used to mobilize pesticides, solvents, and other fat-loving chemicals include:

A. Caloric restriction
B. Sauna therapy
C. Chelation (the technique used to remove heavy metals)

A. **Caloric restriction** is used to mobilize stored toxins from the body and get them back into the bloodstream for metabolism and elimination. Many studies show that decreasing calories—eating less—can mobilize stored toxins. This sounds like a great thing, doesn't it? Just eat less and detoxify. It isn't that simple, though. The studies show that by decreasing calories alone, the toxins do indeed get released from fat stores, but they don't get eliminated from the body and end up getting redistributed to other tissues.[1,2] This is why I never suggest that a person goes on a long fast. Some people think fasting is a great way to detoxify the body. It will definitely cause toxins to be released, but without supporting the liver to break down the toxins and supporting the organs of elimination, the toxins will get redistributed. You can conceivably re-toxify yourself during a fast.

An example of caloric restriction as one part of a cleanse:

♦ Limit calories to 1,000 to 1,500 a day, depending on gender and body size.
♦ Decrease your daily caloric intake by 400-500 calories

B. **Sauna therapy** is also used to mobilize toxins during a detoxification plan. Studies have been conducted using sauna therapy in the U.S. since the 1980s, and sauna therapy has experienced a resurgence since the September 11, 2001 World Trade Center tragedy. After 9/11, many rescue workers and volunteers at Ground Zero started to become ill. Symptoms included difficulty breathing, allergies, headache, fatigue, and more. It is estimated that persons exposed to Ground Zero were exposed to heavy metals, solvents, dioxins, polyaromatic hydrocarbons and other harmful chemicals. Two interesting studies using dry sauna therapy on 9/11 rescue workers show not only its benefits in mobilizing toxins, but also its benefits in increasing elimination of chemicals from the body.

The first study looked at blood levels of PCBs, dioxins and polychlorinated dibenzofurans of seven rescue workers exposed to Ground Zero. They had all had health complaints since working at Ground Zero that ranged from headaches, breathing problems, muscle and joint pain, and skin rashes. They completed a detoxification program using sauna therapy. All seven men had a complete reversal of symptoms, but, more importantly, the chemicals were eliminated from their body. PCB levels declined by 65%, and dioxins and dibenzofurans were below detection limits.[3]

The second study done on 9/11 rescue workers used a specific form of sauna therapy created by L. Ron Hubbard, known as the Hubbard protocol. The results showed a dramatic improvement in symptoms created by exposure to chemicals at Ground Zero.[4] Again, symptoms included respiratory problems such as difficulty breathing, allergies, headache, fatigue, muscle pain and more. The Hubbard protocol includes nutritional supplements to support liver phase-one and phase-two detoxification, polyunsaturated oils, increasing doses of niacin and the use of a sauna. This particular dry sauna protocol involves sweating in a sauna at 140 degrees to 180 degrees for 2.5 to 5 hours with multiple breaks for hydration and cooling-off periods. Numerous studies have been published on the detoxification benefits of the Hubbard sauna protocol.[5,6]

I use one of the following, slightly different, sauna protocols:

♦   10 to 15 minutes in hot dry sauna, not steam room, at 120-140 degrees followed by 30-second cold shower. Repeat 3 to 4 times, and end on cold. Drink electrolyte water during the treatment. I start people off slow in the sauna so they don't release toxins too quickly. Also, some people can be overwhelmed by the heat of the sauna or feel dizzy and faint. Starting with 10-15 minutes heat is very conservative; the goal would be to increase the length of time in the heat during each session, ultimately building up to 30 to 35 minutes of heat.

♦   An alternate method is 30 minutes in an infrared sauna followed by a 30-second cold rinse. Repeat once, end on cold and drink electrolyte water. The cold rinse used here and during the sauna is to remove any toxins excreted on the surface of the skin to prevent them from being reabsorbed.

C. **Chelation** is the method used to mobilize heavy metals from storage sites. Caloric restriction, and sauna therapy can mobilize pesticides, solvents, BPA, phthalates and other chemicals, but heavy metals are tightly bound in the tissue and need a pharmaceutical chelator to get them out ("chelate" means "to bind").

There are three known true chelators used in the U.S.:

♦ DMSA (dimercaptosuccinic acid)
♦ DMPS (2,3-dimercapto-1-propanesulfonic acid)
♦ EDTA (ethylenediaminetetraacetic acid)

In order to mobilize stored heavy metals from the fat tissue, organs or extracellular spaces, there needs to be a pharmaceutical chelator given to mobilize the metals. There are a few over-the-counter supplements that help decrease heavy metal toxicity that you can take if you think you have been exposed to heavy metals. These, of course, are used as part of a comprehensive detoxification plan, outlined below, and not alone.

These include: [7-11]

♦ Selenium
♦ N-acetylcysteine (NAC)
♦ Alpha Lipoic Acid (ALA)
♦ Zinc
♦ Modified citrus pectin

Liver Detoxification

Once the stored toxins are back in the bloodstream, they will reach the liver, where phase-one and phase-two detoxification pathways need to be supported. This is done through food, vitamins, minerals, herbs, amino acids and antioxidants. Liver phase-one detoxification involves making lipid soluble (fat-loving) chemicals more water-soluble. It involves a group of chemical reactions that take place with specific enzymes called the cytochrome P450 enzymes. These chemical reactions are oxidation, reduction, or hydrolysis reactions to add or expose a lipid group to increase water solubility.

Phase-two detoxification then takes the toxin and tries to break it down and make it even more water-soluble so it can be eliminated from the body. Phase-two is a group of pathways where conjugation occurs. This means that something is added to the toxin to help break it down. The main phase-two pathways are methylation, glucaronidation, sulfation, acetylation, and gluathione conjugation.

Remember that some of us are born with genetic alterations in these pathways that make them less efficient. These alterations are called single nucleotide polymorphisms or SNPs. There is a blood test available to determine what SNPs you have in your liver (see the chapter on testing). There are certain herbs, vitamins, amino acids and antioxidants that can improve the function of the SNP.

What about whole foods?

Cruciferous family vegetables, which include cabbage, kale, cauliflower, Brussels sprouts, bok choy, collards, and broccoli, can be used to help liver function. These vegetables contain compounds that help both liver phase-one and phase-two detox pathways.[1] They also help directly break down estrogens in the liver. Another food that should be included in a detoxification plan is beet root. This is good news for those who love beets. Beets increase phase-two detox pathways, which help break down chemicals.[1]

Green tea has so many health benefits that one would be hard-pressed to find a reason not to drink three to four cups a day. Green tea contains a compound called catechins which increases both phase-one and phase-two detoxification. In particular, green tea can increase glutathione, which is an important anti-oxidant for clearing toxins through the liver.[2]

Pomegranate is another drink that can aid detoxification. It contains a compound called ellagic acid, which modulates phase-one cytochrome P450 1A1. This would be a good drink for people born with the genetic polymorphism of 1A1.[2]

Flax seeds are a great source of fiber, which is needed to bind toxins in the bowel and bulk up the stool and decrease constipation. Since toxins are eliminated from the bowel, it is important to have a formed daily bowel movement.

Artichoke has liver protective effects and is an antioxidant.[2] Since most toxins need to be broken down in the liver, any food that can protect the liver should be included in a detoxification plan.

Lastly, *psyllium husk powder* is included for its ability to help eliminate toxins through the bowel, which will be discussed later. It is also a good source of fiber to help decrease constipation and promote a healthy bowel movement. Psyllium husks are from the outer coating of the psyllium seed, like the bran layer of grains.

Foods to include in a detoxification plan are:

- Cruciferous veggies
- Beets
- Green tea
- Pomegranate juice
- Ground flax seeds/meal
- Artichoke
- Psyllium husk powder

What about supplements?

The goal of supplementation during a detoxification plan is to provide nutrients required for liver phase-one and phase-two detox pathways. Herbs that are specific to the liver and gallbladder, called choleretics and cholagogues, are also included. The first required supplement is a quality multivitamin and mineral that can provide the nutrients needed for the enzyme reactions in liver phase-one and phase-two pathways. These are often referred to as "cofactors." These vitamin and mineral cofactors would be taken in a combination product that may also include: green tea and turmeric.

Note: Remember that supplements can interact with prescription medications and with each other so consult a professional first.

Detoxification Cofactors

Here is what to look for in a vitamin and mineral cofactors products:

- Vitamin A (from mixed carotenes)
- Vitamin C
- Vitamins D and E
- All of the B-vitamins

♦ Calcium and magnesium
♦ ′ Zinc and copper
♦ Molybdenum
♦ Kelp and iodine
♦ Selenium
♦ Choline
♦ Inositol
♦ Green tea
♦ Curcumin

Vitamin A is a powerful antioxidant and is also depleted by chlorinated compounds such as organophosphate pesticides and PCBs. The best form is mixed beta carotenes, which is from plants and can be converted in the body to vitamin A.[1,2]

Thiamine is also called vitamin B1. A large amount of thiamine is required because environmental toxins (such as formaldehyde) deplete thiamine. Thiamine is used in liver phase-two detoxification and is needed to restore oxidized glutathione and lipoic acid.[3,4]

Vitamin B6 is needed to clear toxins from the liver. It is needed to process amino acids and neurotransmitters. Chronic exposure to toxins can deplete levels of vitamin B6.[2,4]

Riboflavin, also called vitamin B2, is required for liver phase-one detoxification reactions. It is also a cofactor in glutathione reductase pathways.[2,4]

Magnesium is required because it is often deficient in chemically toxic individuals. Patients who have a high body burden of heavy metals and chemical residue also excrete high amounts of magnesium in their urine. Magnesium is required for cytochrome p450 activity and needed for chemical biotransformation.[4,5]

Selenium increases glutathione peroxidase enzyme levels in the body, which is important in detoxification. It is also a powerful antioxidant for scavenging free radicals.[4]

Molybdenum is a necessary cofactor in liver phase-one and phase-two metabolism.

Kelp is included because it is a concentrated source of minerals, including iodine, magnesium, calcium and potassium.

Iodine is needed to maintain healthy thyroid function, which is often altered due to environmental toxins.[2]

Inositol is required for proper formation of cell membranes and acts as a lipotropic in improving liver functioning.[2,4]

Choline is needed for liver phase-one detoxification reactions and acts as a methyl donor for the synthesis of other compounds.[4]

Green tea is a potent antioxidant. The polyphenols detoxify damaging toxic chemicals. It is shown to prevent the occurrence of cancers, including breast cancer, which is linked to environmental toxins.[6,7]

Curcumin (tumeric) is a plant that has been shown to reduce environmental estrogen induced growth of breast cancer cells.[8] It also increases levels of glutathione in the liver.[8]

Vitamin C is a powerful antioxidant and works synergistically with other anti-oxidants such as glutathione and vitamin E. It increases levels of glutathione in the body.[9]

Vitamin E is a fat soluble vitamin that protects against peroxidation of cell membranes by free radicals. It is an essential antioxidant to fight against toxins in our body.[9]

Niacin is an important cofactor in many biotransformation processes in the body. It is involved in the production of glutathione which is needed for detoxification. It is a cofactor in liver phase 2 sulfation detoxification pathway.[9]

Zinc provides protection against heavy metal toxicity by inhibiting the uptake of lead and cadmium by tissues in the body. Zinc is also a well known antagonist of copper toxicity. Zinc deficiency causes a reduction in glutathione.[9]

Copper – a small amount is added to prevent zinc overload as a strong relationship exists between zinc and copper.[9]

The second supplement to include in a detoxification plan would be an herbal formula that specifically supports the liver and gallbladder. These herbs are often called "choloretics" and "cholagagues." A choloretic is an agent that stimulates the liver to increase output of bile. A cholagogue is an agent that promotes the flow of bile into the intestine, especially as a result of contraction of the gallbladder. It is important during a detoxification plan to dump the bile, which has toxic metabolites, and help eliminate them from the body.

Liver Cleansing Supplements

Example of liver herbs to use during a detoxification plan:

♦ Burdock
♦ Dandelion root
♦ Milk thistle (80% silymarin)
♦ Beet root
♦ Artichoke

Arcticum root, commonly known as burdock, is traditionally used as a blood purifier to clear the bloodstream of toxins. It stimulates bile secretions and aids in detoxification.[1,2]

Taraxacum root, commonly known as dandelion, enhances the flow of bile. It acts on the liver by increasing production and flow of bile to the gallbladder and causes the gallbladder to contract and release stored bile into the intestines. This is why it is considered both a choleretic and a cholagogue.[3]

Silymarin, commonly known as milk thistle, is one of the most well known liver herbs. It is used to treat liver toxicity from organic solvents and to improve liver function tests in numerous liver conditions. Silymarin, the active constituent of milk thistle, causes an alteration of the hepatocyte cell membrane that prevents toxin penetration. It increases glutathione and can scavenge free radicals.[3]

Beet root has antihepatotoxic effects. It is effective against fat deposition in the liver. Beet assists in liver detoxification because it has a high concentration of betaine, which is a methyl donor in the liver's transmethylation pathway.[4,5]

Artichoke is a powerful liver protecting herb that acts as an antioxidant in the liver and protects against chemical toxins. It also increases glutathione levels in the liver cells.[6]

A third supplement that may be included in a detoxification would provide nutrients that help break down estrogens and estrogen mimicking chemicals. Such compounds are linked to conditions like breast cancer, infertility, miscarriage, thyroid dysfunction, endometriosis, fibroids, and menstrual irregularities. To clear these toxins through the liver, a combination of amino acids, antioxidants and nutrients is required to support the liver's detoxification pathways.

Estrogen Detoxification Supplements

Nutrients to include in a cleanse to help hormonal conditions include:

♦ DIM
♦ Calcium-D-Glucarate
♦ NAC
♦ ALA
♦ Methyl B12
♦ Methyl Folate

Diindolylmethane, (DIM), is a metabolite of indole-3-carbonol, I3C. Both increase liver phase-one and phase-two pathways and help metabolize estrogens and chemicals mimicking estrogen. Both are found in cruciferous vegetables like broccoli, Brussels sprouts and cabbage. I3C is converted to diindolylmethane in the stomach. Both I3C and DIM alter urinary estrogen metabolite profiles in women. DIM can regulate and promote a more efficient metabolism of estrogen.[1,2]

Calcium-D-Glucarate is a substance naturally produced by humans and is also found in fruits and vegetables, particularly the cruciferous family vegetables. It has the ability to increase glucuronidation, an enzyme pathway in liver phase-two detoxification necessary for excretion of toxic compounds. Calcium-D-Glucarate also inhibits the enzyme beta-glucuronidase, allowing the body to excrete estrogen before it can be reabsorbed and raise serum levels of estrogen.[3,4]

N-Acetyl Cysteine (NAC) is a powerful antioxidant with rapid oral absorption. It is the precursor to L-cysteine and reduced glutathione (GSH). NAC promotes liver detoxification by restoring glutathione levels in the body. It also protects against environmental toxins by scavenging reactive oxygen species. NAC can increase the metabolism of estrogen through the liver.[5,6,7]

Alpha Lipoic Acid (ALA) is a powerful antioxidant that scavenges reactive oxygen species protecting against oxidative damage caused by environmental toxins. ALA induces liver phase-two detoxification enzymes and specifically stimulates glutathione synthesis. ALA is effective in removing heavy metals from the body by itself and when combined with DMSA. It can promote clearance of estrogens in the liver by increasing the phase-two glutathione pathway.[5,8]

Methylcobalamin (vitamin B12) and Methylfolate (folic acid) are naturally occurring substances in the body. Each of these consists of a methyl group that, when metabolized in the body, cleaves off and increases methylation. Methylation is part of liver phase-two metabolism and is responsible for breaking down estrogens. By supporting methylation pathways, you promote detoxification of estrogens and environmental estrogens. [9,10,11]

These are just a few of the supplements to be considered during a detoxification plan. There are many others that can increase the liver's ability to break down toxic compounds. Not every herb or nutrient listed is necessary for every individual. Please know that some herbs and nutrients can interact with medication and a doctor should be consulted if you're taking supplements while on prescription medications. I always tell my patients that anyone can react negatively to anything. So just because it is natural or because you can buy it over the counter at a health food store doesn't always mean it is safe. If you ever have a bad reaction to a supplement, stop taking it immediately and call your doctor.

Let's get it out

Once the liver finishes breaking down the toxin and creating a water-soluble byproduct, it needs to get eliminated. This occurs through the bowel, kidney, skin and lungs. Deep breathing, meditation and exercise are always included in a detoxification plan to promote healthy and normal breathing patterns. Sauna therapy, used earlier to help release the stored toxin, is also used to help get the broken-down byproduct out through the skin. It is important to drink plenty of fluids during the day to help flush toxins out through the kidneys. But how much water should you drink each day? It is recommended to drink half your body weight in ounces of filtered water a day. Other forms of water therapy, known as hydrotherapy, are also used to increase circulation of the blood and lymph to get the toxins through the kidney or to promote sweating.

Elimination of toxins occurs through:

A. Hydrotherapy- showers, baths and constitutional hydrotherapy
B. Bowel support- castor oil packs, colonics and coffee enemas

A. **Hydrotherapy** refers to the use of water to treat disease, or, better explained, it is the application of alternating hot and cold on the body to have a therapeutic effect. Sauna therapy was described earlier as a means of mobilizing toxins. As you recall, the form of sauna therapy described did involve alternating hot and cold (10 to 15 minutes in the hot sauna followed by a 30-second cold shower). This is repeated 4 to 5 times and should be done several times in a week. Not only does this release stored toxins, but the heat creates perspiration on the skin, which is a way to excrete toxins. In order for the toxins to not be reabsorbed through the skin, the cold shower is used to rinse off the skin and clear any toxins excreted through perspiration in the sauna. As I mentioned earlier, I start patients off with only 10 to 15 minutes in the sauna followed by a cold rinse with the goal of increasing the amount of time in the heat to 30 to 40 minutes, followed by a cold rinse.

Other forms of hydrotherapy exist as well, and under the same principle of alternating hot and cold, can be used to help increase circulation of the blood and lymph system to move toxins to the organs of elimination. Remember that the organs of elimination include the kidney and bowel. The use of heat is done in brief periods of time, (less than 15 minutes). The short application of heat causes an increase in circulation whereas long applications of heat cause a decrease in circulation.[1]

So what forms of hydrotherapy can be done at home?

1. Alternating hot and cold shower: 3 minutes of a hot shower, 30 seconds of a cold shower; repeat 3 times and end on cold.

2. Epsom salt bath: 10-minute hot bath with 1 cup of Epsom salt; end with a 1-minute cold shower.

3. Constitutional Hydrotherapy Treatment is a very old and traditional naturopathic therapy involving the use of water as therapy. Typically, a physician performs the treatment in his or her office. It typically involves placing hot and cold towels on the body and uses an electrical modality called a sine-wave machine. This traditional therapy can be altered and performed at home as a way to get the blood and lymphatic system moving throughout the body. This movement of blood and lymph during a cleanse helps bring toxins to the organs of metabolism (liver) and elimination (kidney). Constitutional hydrotherapy promotes detoxification, improves nutrition, and increases immunity.[1]

Home application of constitutional hydrotherapy

Contraindications: Persons with acute asthma, acute infections, or low temperature (< 97°F oral) should not perform constitutional hydrotherapy.

Caution: Avoid becoming chilled. If feeling chilly, add more blankets or place a hot water bottle or other heat source over the feet.

Supplies:
Shower or Bath	4 Towels
2 Blankets	1 Sheet

Directions:

1. Spread two blankets lengthwise on a bed with a sheet over them. The person to be treated should lie on his or her back, unclothed from the hips up.

2. Thoroughly wring out two towels in hot water and place onto the chest and abdomen.

3. Wrap the sheet and blankets tightly around the body and leave in place for five minutes.

4. Wring out one towel in hot water and another in cold water.

5. Replace the towels on the chest and abdomen with the hot towel.

6. Place the cold towel on top of the hot one. Flip these over, leaving the cold one on the chest and abdomen.

7. Again, wrap the sheet and blankets tightly around the body and leave in place for at least ten minutes.

8. Then rest. You may sleep, use visualization, or meditate during this time.

9. Remove the towel when it is warm to the touch.

10. Repeat this procedure with the person lying on his or her stomach and apply towels to the back. Rest and leave in place for at least ten minutes.

B. **Bowel Support.** Next the bowel needs to be supported to promote a normal formed daily bowel movement and promote the secretion and excretion of bile from the liver and gallbladder. This is done through the use of castor oil packs, colon hydrotherapy and coffee enemas. Increasing dietary fiber is important to maintain a formed and healthy daily bowel movement. Adding 2 tablespoons of ground flax seeds a day to the diet will accomplish this goal.

1. A castor oil pack is something that is applied to the skin, typically over the liver, which is located on the right side of the upper abdomen just under the lower ribs, and over the lower abdomen where the bowel is located. Castor oil has a long history of traditional medical use, dating back to ancient Egypt. Derived from the castor bean (Ricinus Communis), the oil was once used internally as a laxative but is now primarily used externally due to its potential toxicity. A castor oil pack is placed on the skin to increase circulation and to promote elimination. It is used to stimulate the liver, increase lymphatic circulation, reduce inflammation, and improve digestion.[2,3]

How to make a castor oil pack

Castor oil packs are made by applying a small amount of castor oil to a piece of flannel and placing it on the skin. The flannel is covered with a towel, and then a hot water bottle or heating pad is placed over the towel to heat the pack.

A castor oil pack can be placed on the following body regions:

♦ The right side of the abdomen to stimulate the liver.
♦ The abdomen to relieve constipation and other digestive disorders.
♦ The uterus for uterine fibroids and other disorders.

Castor oil should not be taken internally. It should not be applied to broken skin, or used during pregnancy, breastfeeding, or during menstrual flow.

Materials:

♦ Undyed wool or cotton flannel large enough to cover the affected area
♦ Castor oil
♦ Towel
♦ Hot water bottle
♦ Container with lid or zip-lock bag
♦ Old clothes and sheets (castor oil will stain clothing and bedding)

Directions:

1. Place a small amount of oil on one side of the flannel and rub it in.

2. Place the pack over the affected body part.
3. Cover with a towel.
4. Place the hot water bottle over the pack. Leave it on for 30 to 60 minutes.
5. After removing the pack, cleanse the area with water and baking soda.
6. Store the pack in the zip-lock bag or container in the refrigerator.

2. Colon hydrotherapy is also used to help remove toxins from the body by providing support to the organs of elimination; they promote bile dumping and relieve constipation. Colonics are administered by trained and certified colon hydrotherapists in a clinic setting. Their purpose is to infuse water into the entire colon, which is then released through an enclosed system which clears compounds dumped from the liver into the intestines. Water temperature and pressure are closely monitored in a series of fills and releases. Colonics are included in a detoxification plan for the elimination of toxins from the body via the primary active excretion of bile.[4] The benefits of colonics have been debated for years in this country. Conventional medicine typically thinks colonics are useless and possibly dangerous while alternative medicine cites examples of numerous conditions helped by colon hydrotherapy.[5,6] Even in conventional medicine, colon hydrotherapy has been used to treat fecal incontinence. [7]

Some people are not good candidates for colon hydrotherapy due to a lack of colon (bowel resection), rectal prolapsed, pain, polyps, colon cancer, ulcerative colitis, Crohn's disease (in the acute inflammatory stages), severe hemorrhoids, or a tumor in the rectum or large intestine. Make sure your doctor clears you for colon hydrotherapy by taking a good medical history and performing an anoscopic exam. Some people are hesitant to get a colonic or don't know how to find a good colon hydrotherapist. Make sure you find someone who is properly trained and certified to explain the procedure in depth.

This is information I give my patients about colonics. This was developed by the National College of Natural Medicine in Portland Oregon (*www.ncnm.edu*).

What are "Colonics?"

Colonic hydrotherapy uses water to gently cleanse the large intestine or colon. Colonics are used to cleanse the body of toxins that build up in the colon. Sometimes these toxins can no longer be effectively eliminated through the large intestine due to problems in the bowel. Colonics also promote the release of toxic bile.

What do studies on colonics tell us?

♦ Increased amounts of toxic bile and lymph, chlorinated pesticides and heavy metals are released; and
♦ These levels exceed the levels that are cleared with daily BMs.

What to look for in a Colon Therapist:

♦ Knowledgeable about toxicity and cleansing
♦ Trained in proper clearance techniques
♦ Most colon therapists don't understand how colonics relate to environmental medicine, so follow your physicians' orders
♦ You need to find out what their typical protocol is and how they feel about frequency of sessions
♦ Proper sanitary precautions/sterilization
♦ Sterilization of machine and table

♦ Filtered water
♦ Adequate ventilation and exhaust fans
♦ Available bathroom close by

What to Expect at your First Visit

You will be lying comfortably on your back on the treatment table as the therapist administers the colonic. Your only job is to relax as much as possible and remember to breathe! The colonics should never be painful–the most discomfort will probably be some cramping, somewhat like you would experience with diarrhea.

Some people complain of a slightly "toxic" feeling after their first treatment. This is most likely due to the toxins that can get stirred up and reabsorbed into the bloodstream. To eliminate these toxins, drink several glasses of water throughout the day after the initial treatment and follow your physicians' post-colonic recommendations.

What Should I Eat Before/After the Colonic?

My recommendation is to do what is most comfortable for you. Many people find that eating only lightly before or after the colonic, or even fasting the day of the treatment, helps them feel that the cleanse has been more complete.

How Often Should I Have a Colonic?

Opinions on this vary widely. I prescribe colonics for the purpose of removing toxic products from the bowel and bile. The treatments are often timed with heavy metal chelation or used with a detoxification plan. Treatments are individualized and the number depends on how strong your vital force is and how many toxins might be stored in your body. Follow your physicians' prescription. After having a series of treatments, you will know what it feels like to detoxify.

What do we expect to see?

♦ Often it will take 2 to 3 colonics before the body will start to dump toxic bile
♦ Some very toxic people dump high amounts with the first colonic.
♦ Bile dumps (yellow/orange/red)
♦ Lymph Releases (billowy white)
♦ Heavy metal releases (sand on bottom of tube)
♦ Mucus
♦ Food particles
♦ Some fecal material
♦ You cannot see yeast (candida) coming out of a colonic.

About Acidophilus

During the colonic, many harmful toxins are washed out of the colon. At the same time, helpful bacteria, including Lactobacillus acidophilus, are removed. It is important to replace the healthful bacteria to restore the natural, healthy balance of the intestinal flora. I recommend taking a supplement with high amounts of L. acidophilus and Bifido bacterium with each meal for up to one week after the colonic.

3. A coffee enema is another method used to help eliminate toxins through the bowel and promote a normal bowel release. This is an option for those who can't get colon hydrotherapy due to medical issues or cost. An enema only stimulates the first part of the colon, the sigmoid colon, and does not cleanse the entire colon as a colonic does. Enemas have been used in conventional medicine for years to clear the sigmoid colon

prior to a procedure called a sigmiodoscopy. Coffee enemas were made popular in the U.S. by Max Gerson, of the infamous Gerson therapy for cancer (which is really a detoxification protocol). Studies have shown that coffee enemas cause dilation of the bile ducts, which facilitates excretion of toxic byproducts in the bowel.[8] They also have been shown to increase liver phase-two glutathione pathway.[8] Caffeine enemas facilitate excretion of toxic breakdown products by the liver and dialysis of toxic products from across the colonic wall.[9]

After being cleared by your doctor of any anal, rectal or sigmoid colon disease, a coffee enema can be performed at home. There are many different methods on how to prepare coffee and administer it in an enema.

Here is one example from *www.ineedcoffee.com*:

You will need to buy a re-usable enema kit. Enema products are available at many stores. They are usually disposable and are inexpensive.

Supplies:
- ◆ Organic coffee (any roasting level will do)
- ◆ French press pot
- ◆ Filtered water

Recipe:

1. Bring 8 cups of water to a boil.
2. Grind eight heaping spoonfuls of organic coffee. Put it in a French press pot. You can use a drip coffee maker, but be sure to use organic, non-bleached coffee filters.
3. Pour the water over the coffee grounds and let it steep, then cool for one hour or more.

4. After this amount of time, the liquid should be about body temperature. If you stick your finger in the water, it should be lukewarm or cool, but not hot.
5. Press the coffee grounds to the bottom, then pour the coffee liquid into the enema bag.
6. Never utilize flavored coffee, sweetened coffee, or coffee with milk (cafe au lait) for this purpose.

Directions:

Make sure to use an at-home enema or colonic kit that includes a bag that is sturdy enough to accept lukewarm coffee. Make sure that there are no grounds in the enema bag or enema hose; also ensure that the hose doesn't get a kink in it. Follow the directions that accompany the enema kit you purchased. Lie on your right side, inject and attempt to retain the coffee for 10 to 15 minutes. Change positions while retaining the coffee. After a few minutes turn over onto your back, a few minutes later, switch to your left side before evacuating your bowels. Most people lie in the bathtub to perform the enema in order to hang the bag from someplace high such as the showerhead and to be close to the toilet when it is time to evacuate the bowels.

Supporting the organs of elimination can be accomplished by:

♦ Hydrotherapy (sauna, constitutional hydrotherapy, and showers and baths)
♦ Increasing dietary fiber
♦ Castor oil packs
♦ Colon hydrotherapy
♦ Coffee enema
♦ Drinking half your body weight in ounces of filtered water each day

Summary

Now that I have broken down each component of a detoxification plan, let's put it all together. It is important to first see your physician to make sure your liver, kidneys, and lungs are free of disease and functioning properly. Colonics cannot be performed if you have the contraindications mentioned above. This detoxification plan can be individualized based on your preferred form of hydrotherapy, access to a sauna or colon hydrotherapy, or based on your SNPs if you had them tested. If you have heavy metals in your body, then a chelation protocol would be added to the plan by your physician. Proper chelating agents include DMSA, DMPS and EDTA. These are typically administered either orally or intravenously.

Remember: the four steps in a detoxification plan are:

♦ Mobilize stored toxins
♦ Support liver metabolism
♦ Support elimination
♦ Avoid exposure to toxins in the environment

8 Weeks to Women's Wellness

Sample 8-week detoxification plan

A. Nutrition

♦ Eat 3 to 4 servings of cruciferous family veggies a day.
♦ Eat 2 tbsp. Bob's Red Mill ground flax seed/meal a day on food.
♦ Take 2 tsp. psyllium husk powder a day in water.
♦ Drink 3 to 4 cups a day of green tea or red roobios tea if sensitive to caffeine.
♦ Add beets and artichoke to your diet.
♦ Drink 6 ounces of pomegranate juice each day.

- No red meat, no sugar, no coffee, no alcohol and no dairy.
- If you eat fish low it must be fish low in mercury.
- 1 to 2 servings of whole grains are okay, but must be organic.
- Turkey and chicken are okay, but must be organic.
- Fruits and legumes are ok to eat, but must be organic.
- Decrease your daily caloric intake by 300 calories unless you are underweight.

B. Hydrotherapy/cleansing

- Sauna therapy (15 minutes hot, 30-second cold rinse, repeat and end on cold). This should be a 45-minute treatment and performed 3 to 4 times a week. Try to increase the time in the heat to 30 minutes.
  Caution: If you had lymph nodes removed for breast cancer, the heat of a sauna may be contraindicated.
- Alternating hot/cold shower (3 minutes hot, 30 seconds cold; repeat and end on cold).
- Castor oil packs daily over uterus and liver (30 minutes with heat except during menses).
- Colonics (2 a week for 4 weeks for the last 4 weeks of the 2-month cleanse, if cleared by your doctor).

C. Supplements by Health Freedom Nutrition www.hfn-usa.com

- Detox Cofactors™ (6 caps a day)
- Estro Relief™ (3 caps a day)
- Hepa Cleanse™ (2 caps a day)

Before taking any supplements, check with your doctor for drug-herb interactions. These are from the detoxification line from Health Freedom Nutrition (www.hfn-usa.com), which I formulated. However, you may use any manufacturer that has the herbs, vitamins, minerals and nutrients discussed above.

Caution: If you have cancer wait until you complete chemotherapy or radiation to take these supplements.

D. Avoidance

Read the chapter on avoiding chemicals in your everyday life to prevent re-exposure.

If trying to conceive, at the end of the 8-week detoxification plan, consider a product to support the uterus to get ready for pregnancy. One such product is called Pregnancy Prep by Vitanica, and consists of tribulus terrestris extract, rhodiola rosea extract, chaste tree berry extract, raspberry leaf, alfalfa leaf, dong quai, motherwort leaf, and unicorn root.

If you have PCOS and finish the 8-week detoxification plan, then consider a supplement to control sugar cravings and lower insulin resistance, as this is often a component to PCOS. Such a product may consist of chromium, vanadium, holy basil, bitter melon, panax ginseng, cinnamon, magnesium. Also consider a supplement to lower testosterone, which is often elevated in PCOS. This may consist of nettles root, green tea, saw palmetto, sarsaparilla, bloodroot.

If you have been tested for heavy metals through blood or urine testing and have elevated levels, then a chelating agent will need to be added to your plan by your physician. The colonic portion of the plan will change and will be timed with the type of chelator being prescribed.

CHAPTER VII
TO SUM IT ALL UP

You now know more than most as to why so many women have health problems related to hormone disrupting chemicals in the environment. You also know what can be done to prevent these health problems and reverse them. How are you going to use this information to get yourself well? How are you going to make changes in your life to keep yourself healthy? Are you going to tell others what you have learned? Are you going to call for action to get these chemicals out of our environment?

Some of this information can be overwhelming, and you may not know where to begin. It obviously begins with some major lifestyle changes. Keep in mind that this doesn't have to happen all at once. Some may be too sick and need to start simply with diet changes. Some may be going through chemotherapy or radiation for breast cancer and need to wait a while to start the supplements. Some may be so gung-ho that they go out and purchase a sauna for their home, clean out their kitchen of all plastics and dive right into a detoxification plan.

Some of you may already have known most of the information in this book, and for others it is going to be similar to learning a new language.

I suggest starting with an outline:

1. Get organized
2. Make time for yourself
3. Clean up your diet
4. Clean up your air
5. Clean up your water
6. Get rid of the chemicals in your home
7. Consider your genes, consider getting tested
8. Listen to your body
9. Get into the sauna
10. Go easy on the supplements

1. Get organized
Re-read through the parts of this book that was the most important or meaningful to you. Write out your plan. Your plan may start by simply getting a filter for your bedroom, or it may begin with changing what you eat. You may copy the sections of this book that outline simply avoidance techniques, or the 8-week detoxification plan. Are you interested in a detoxification plan to treat a certain health problem or prevent one? Are you out to change your diet or the products you buy? Is it time to start exercising? Is it time to make an appointment with a licensed naturopathic doctor? (See *www.naturopathic.org* to find a physician in your area.)

2. Make time for yourself
Women are mothering and nurturing by nature. The problem is that we nurture everyone but ourselves. It is now time for you to focus on you. Doctor's orders.

If you aren't healthy in mind, body and spirit, then you can't be of use to anyone else, including yourself. Eight weeks isn't that long. Eight weeks is your time for you.

3. Clean up your diet

Eat organic fruits and vegetables, meat and dairy products. Get rid of the plastic bottles, food storage containers, and plastic wrap. Start to introduce foods from the diet section of the detoxification plan.

4. Clean up your air

Get a room HEPA air filter.

5. Clean up your water

Get a water filter for the home and avoid plastic water bottles.

6. Get rid of the chemicals in your home

Re-read the avoidance section of this book and avoid chemicals in your cleaning, grooming, and beauty products.

7. Consider your genes

I mentioned several times that your genetic make-up could be the reason you don't automatically detoxify these chemicals. Consider getting tested for single nucleotide polymorphisms, SNPs. Think about the women in your family. What conditions have they had that are hormonally driven? This is often a predictor or explanation of your health.

8. Listen to your body

After being in the health care field for 20 years and working primarily with women's health conditions, I have learned to listen to a woman when she says, "My hormones are out of balance." Listen to yourself. Trust your intuition and seek out medical advice.

9. Get into the sauna

This treatment is outlined in the chapter on treatment, and is the easy place to begin to remove chemicals from the body.

10. Go easy on the supplements

Just because it is sold over the counter at a grocery store or sold on the Internet doesn't mean it is safe. Many supplements contain herbs and nutrients that can interact with each other and with prescription medication. If you are taking a prescription medication, see your doctor before taking any supplements. There is no magic pill, prescription or supplement. It starts with diet, exercise, lifestyle changes, and education on avoidance.

A call to action

Removing chemicals from the body that should never be there in the first place seems like an unnecessary thing that we should not have to do. Avoiding chemicals in the food, air, water and products we use is not something my grandmother had to deal with in her lifetime. This book has armed you with knowledge not only to improve your health but also to improve the health of the planet. I ask you to get involved. Demand that legislators improve the air quality where you live, remove harmful chemicals from the water, place restrictions on industry in your state, protect the food supply and regulate cosmetics, cleaning products and household goods.

Some resources where you can learn more include:

1. Breast Cancer Action - *www.bcaction.org*

A membership organization that advocates for policy changes directed at the prevention of breast cancer and the development of safer, more effective treatments.

2. Breast Cancer Fund - *www.breastcancerfund.org*
A nonprofit organization that identifies and advocates for the elimination of the environmental causes of breast cancer. Provides reports and fact sheets on chemicals and breast cancer.

3. Collaborative on Health and the Environment - *www.healthandenvironment.org and www.database.healthandenvironment.org/*
A network of more than 3,000 individuals and organizations working to address growing concerns about the links between human health and environmental factors. The Toxicant and Disease Database summarizes links between chemical contaminants and 180 human diseases.

4. The Endocrine Disruption Exchange - *www.endocrinedisruption.com*
A nonprofit organization that compiles scientific evidence on the health and environmental problems caused by exposure to chemicals that interfere with hormones, with a special focus on development.

5. Environmental Health News - *www.environmentalhealthnews.org*
A syndication service that is published daily by Environmental Health Sciences. It both publishes its own articles and offers summaries of articles published in referenced journals as well as a daily digest of articles on environmental health topics.

6. Pesticide Action Network, North America - *www.panna.org and www.pesticideinfo.org/*
A nonprofit organization that promotes the elimination of highly hazardous pesticides and offers a pesticide database on toxicity and regulatory information, including data on pesticide use in California.

7. Silent Spring Institute - *www.silentspring.org and www. silentspring.org/sciencereview*
A partnership of scientists, physicians, public-health advocates, and community activists that works to identify the links between the environment and women's health, especially breast cancer. Silent Spring Institute provides a database on the 216 different chemicals shown to cause mammary gland cancer in animals, including individual study results, chemical regulatory status, and likely sources of exposure.

Parting words

Health and the environment are not independent of each other, as some may believe. Women are exposed to more chemicals in their daily lives than ever before. These chemicals not only harm the planet, but also your health. Removing chemicals from the body is restoring wellness. Avoiding the toxins in the environment is maintaining wellness. Keeping chemicals out of the food, air, water and products in the first place is the key to wellness.

Your health is in your hands. It is a package deal. Educate yourself on how you are exposed to chemicals, take steps to avoid those chemicals, learn which specific chemical is linked to a hormonal condition you have or are at risk of getting, and begin to cleanse and detoxify. This will start you on the road to health and wellness.

RESOURCES

Websites

www.drmarchese.com

Marianne Marchese ND, LLC is a clinician, author, and educator. She graduated from Creighton University in 1990 with a B.S. in Occupational Therapy and specialized in neurological and orthopedic conditions. Dr. Marchese received her Doctorate of Naturopathic Medicine from the National College of Naturopathic Medicine (NCNM) in Portland Oregon. She completed a two-year postgraduate residency in Integrative Medicine and Women's Health and completed a six-month post-graduate training in Environmental Medicine.

Dr. Marchese has been in private practice and an adjunct faculty member at a post-graduate college since 2002. She first taught at the National College of Naturopathic Medicine and later at Life Chiropractic College. Currently, she is professor of Gynecology at the Southwest College of Naturopathic Medicine in Tempe, AZ. Dr. Marchese maintains a private practice in Phoenix AZ, and is frequently interviewed by local and national media for her expertise in women's health and environmental medicine and was named in *Phoenix* Magazines' 2010 Top Doctor Issue as one of the top naturopathic physicians in the Phoenix metropolitan area.

Dr. Marchese has had articles and quotes published in magazines and journals such as: *Better Nutrition Magazine, Raising Arizona Kids Magazine, Taste for Life Magazine, Townsend Letter and Symbiosis Journal*, the *Journal of Natural Medicine*, and more. She is a well recognized speaker and has presented at the American Association of Naturopathic Physicians Convention, American College for Advancement of Medicine, Arizona Naturopathic Medical Association Convention, Canadian Association of Naturopathic Doctors Convention, iMosaic Conference, The Institute for Women's Health and Integrative Medicine, California and Washington Naturopathic Physician state conference, The International College of Integrative Medicine and San Francisco State University and more.

Dr. Marchese currently has a bi-monthly column on environmental medicine in *The Townsend Letter*.

Dr. Marchese has served on the legislative committee for the California Naturopathic Doctors Association, is past Vice President of the Arizona Naturopathic Medical Association and currently is on the board of directors for the Council of Naturopathic Medical Education.

www.8weekstowomenswellness.com

The official site for *8 Weeks to Women's Wellness* by Dr. Marianne Marchese.

www.smart-publications.com

Smart Publications
P.O. Box 4667
Petaluma, CA 94955
800-976-2783
email: admin@smart-publications.com

Smart Publications publishes health and nutrition information. Their mission is to "Clarify the Complex World of Nutrition Science." Their newsletter, Smart Publications *Health & Wellness Update* is mailed to 50,000 subscribers each month and their website provides a wealth of information on the subject of nutrition and alternative health. The book publishing arm has published top titles by medical experts like Dr. Garry Gordon and Dr. Jonathan V. Wright. *8 Weeks to Women's Wellness* by Dr. Marianne Marchese is the most recent book from Smart Publications.

www.ewg.org

Environmental Working Group
1436 U Street. NW, Suite 100
Washington, DC 20009
202-667-6982
Skin deep-cosmetic safety database – safe sunscreen list – pesticides on food and mercury in fish lists

The mission of the Environmental Working Group (EWG) is to use the power of public information to protect public health and the environment. Their research brings to light unsettling facts that you have a right to know. It shames and shakes up polluters and their lobbyists. It rattles politicians and shapes policy. It persuades bureaucracies to rethink science and strengthen regulation. It provides practical information you can use to protect your family and community.

www.womenandenvironment.org

Women's Voices for the Earth
114 W Pine St – PO Box 8743
Missoula, MT 59807
406-543-3747
email: womensvoices@womensvoices.org

Women's Voices for the Earth is a national organization that works to eliminate toxic chemicals that impact women's health by changing consumer behaviors, corporate practices and government policies.

Their vision is a world in which all women have the right to live in a healthy environment, free from toxic chemicals that adversely impact their health and well-being. Women will be leaders in this world, where corporate practices and government policies ensure that the water they drink, the food they eat, the air they breathe, and the products they use in their homes and workplaces are not contaminated with toxic chemicals that may impact their health.

www.when.org

Women's Health & Environmental Network (WHEN)
704 North 23rd Street
Philadelphia, PA 19130
215-990-1271
email: info@when.org

We have a responsibility for the stewardship of our health and our planet to protect against contamination from chemicals, pesticides, and toxic waste through a toxin-free, clean environment.

In recognizing the nexus between health and environment, the Women's Health & Environmental Network (WHEN) is dedicated to:

- ◆ Educating about this interrelationship;
- ◆ Researching the effects of this link upon women and their families;
- ◆ Advocating for policies that minimize or eliminate the exposure of harmful substances at the local, state and federal levels;
- ◆ Developing responses to minimize harm to health and the environment.

www.nottoopretty.org

The Campaign for Safe Cosmetics
email: info@safecosmetics.org

The Campaign for Safe Cosmetics is a coalition effort launched in 2004 to protect the health of consumers and workers by securing the corporate, regulatory and legislative reforms necessary to eliminate dangerous chemicals from cosmetics and personal care products.

Key nonprofit coalition partners in the Campaign include the Alliance for a Healthy Tomorrow (represented by Clean Water Action and Massachusetts Breast Cancer Coalition), the Breast Cancer Fund, Commonweal, Environmental Working Group, Friends of the Earth and Women's Voices for the Earth. The Breast Cancer Fund, a national 501(c)(3) organization focused on preventing breast cancer by identifying and eliminating the environmental links to the disease, serves as the national coordinator for the Campaign.

They are working with more than 100 endorsing organizations, thousands of grassroots supporters and over 1,300 companies that have signed the Compact for Safe Cosmetics.

www.ehponline.com

Environmental Health Perspectives
c/o Brogan & Partners
14600 Weston Parkway
Cary, NC 27513
919-653-2581

Environmental Health Perspectives (EHP) provides free full-text journal articles on environmental medicine. *EHP* is a monthly journal of peer-reviewed research and news published by the U.S. National Institute of Environmental Health Sciences, National Institutes of Health, Department of Health and Human Services. *EHP*'s mission is to serve as a forum for the discussion of the interrelationships between the environment and human health by publishing in a balanced and objective manner the best peer-reviewed research and most current and credible news of the field. With an impact factor of 6.19, *EHP* is the top monthly journal in public, environmental, and occupational health and the second-ranked monthly journal in environmental sciences.

The environmental health sciences include many fields of study and increasingly comprise a multidisciplinary research area. *EHP* publishes articles from a wide range of scientific disciplines encompassing basic research; epidemiologic studies; risk assessment; relevant ethical, legal, social, environmental justice, and policy topics; longitudinal human studies; in vitro and in vivo animal research with a clear relationship to human health; and environmental medicine case reports. Because children are uniquely sensitive to their environments, *EHP* devotes a research section specifically to issues surrounding children's environmental health.

www.scorecard.org

Scorecard – The Pollution Information website.
Green Media Toolshed
1800 M Street, NW
Suite 300 North
Washington, DC 20036
(202) 659-7710

Scorecard is the web's most popular resource for information about pollution problems and toxic chemicals. Find out about the pollution problems in your community and learn who is responsible. See which geographic areas and companies have the worst pollution records. Identify which racial/ethnic and income groups bear more than their share of environmental burdens. Then take action as an informed citizen—you can fax a polluting company, contact your elected representatives, or get involved in your community.

www.atsdr.cdc.gov

Agency for Toxic Substances and Disease Registry
4770 Buford Hwy NE
Atlanta, GA 30341
800-232-4636
email: cdcinfo@cdc.gov

The Agency for Toxic Substances and Disease Registry (ATSDR), based in Atlanta, Georgia, is a federal public health agency of the U.S. Department of Health and Human Services. ATSDR serves the public by using the best science, taking responsive public health actions, and providing trusted health information to prevent harmful exposures and diseases related to toxic substances.

www.healthandenvironment.org

The Collaborative on Health and the Environment
c/o Commonweal, PO Box 316
Bolinas, CA 94924
email: info@healthandenvironment.org

The Collaborative on Health and the Environment (CHE) is an international partnership committed to strengthening the scientific and public dialogue on the impact of environmental factors on human health and catalyzing initiatives to address these concerns. CHE has been instrumental in leveraging mainstream health-affected constituencies in the environmental health science revolution and engaging researchers, health professionals, and environmental health and justice advocates from diverse sectors. Founded in 2002, CHE is an international partnership of over 3,500 individuals and organizations in 45 countries and 48 states, including scientists, health professionals, health-affected groups, non-governmental organizations and other concerned citizens, committed to improving human and ecological health.

www.environmentalhealthnews.org

Environmental Health News
Environmental Health Sciences
421 Park St., Ste. 4
Charlottesville, Virginia 22902
434-220-0348

This site allows you to subscribe to a daily email newsletter keeping you up-to-date on what is happening in the environment. The mission of Environmental Health News is to advance the public's understanding of environmental health issues by publishing its own journalism and providing access to worldwide news about a variety of subjects related to the health of humans, wildlife and ecosystems.

www.beyondpesticides.org

Beyond Pesticides
701 E Street, SE, Suite 200
Washington, DC 20003
202-543-5450
email: info@beyondpesticides.org

Beyond Pesticides provides the public with useful information on pesticides and alternatives to their use. With this information, people can and do protect themselves and the environment from the potential adverse public health and environmental effects associated with the use and misuse of pesticides.

www.noharm.org

Health Care Without Harm
1901 N. Moore Street, Suite 509
Arlington, VA 22209
703-243-0056

"First Do No Harm" ... Together with our partners around the world, Health Care Without Harm shares a vision of a health care sector that does no harm, and instead promotes the health of people and the environment.

To that end, we are working to implement ecologically sound and healthy alternatives to health care practices that pollute the environment and contribute to disease.

Books

What's in this stuff? by Patricia Thomas
> Perigee Trade; 1 edition (January 2, 2008)
> ISBN-10: 0399533885

Drop-Dead Gorgeous: Protecting Yourself from the Hidden Dangers of Cosmetics by Kim Erickson
> McGraw-Hill; 1 edition (March 4, 2002)
> ISBN-10: 0658017934 ISBN-13: 978-0658017933

Our Stolen Future: Are We Threatening Our Fertility, Intelligence, and Survival?— A Scientific Detective Story
> by Theo Colburn, Dianne Dumanoski, John Peter Meyers
> Plume (March 1, 1997)
> ISBN-10: 0452274141   ISBN-13: 978-0452274143

Living Downstream: An Ecologist's Personal Investigation of Cancer and the Environment by Sandra Steingraber
> Da Capo Press; Second Edition, Revised and updated edition (March 23, 2010)
> ISBN-10: 0306818698   ISBN-13: 978-0306818691

A Consumer's Dictionary of Household, Yard and Office Chemicals: Complete Information About Harmful and Desirable Chemicals Found in Everyday Home Products, Yard Poisons, and Office Polluters by Ruth Winter
> ASJA Press (August 2, 2007)
> ISBN-10: 0595449484 ISBN-13: 978-0595449484

Women's Encyclopedia of Natural Medicine: Alternative Therapies and Integrative Medicine for Total Health and Wellness
> by Tori Hudson
> McGraw-Hill; 2 edition (September 20, 2007)
> ISBN-10: 0071464735 ISBN-13: 978-0071464734

The Definitive Guide to Cancer, 3rd Edition: An Integrative Approach to Prevention, Treatment, and Healing
> by Lise Alschuler, Karolyn A. Gazella
> Celestial Arts; 3 edition (April 27, 2010)
> ISBN-10: 1587613581 ISBN-13: 978-1587613586

The Breast Cancer Companion by Barb McDonald
> *www.thebreastcancercompanion.com*

Clean Green and Lean; Remove Toxins that Make you Fat
> by Walter Crinnion
> Wiley; 1 edition (March 1, 2010)
> ISBN-10: 0470409231 ISBN-13: 978-0470409237

The GenoType Diet: Change Your Genetic Destiny to Live the Longest, Fullest, and Healthiest Life Possible
> by Peter D'Adamo
> Crown Archetype; First Edition edition
> (December 26, 2007)
> ISBN-10: 0767925246 ISBN-13: 978-0767925242

Enhancing Fertility: A Couple's Guide to Natural Approaches
> by Chris Meletis and Liz Brown
> Basic Health Publications; 1 edition (May 2004)
> ISBN-10: 1591200547 ISBN-13: 978-1591200543

Green home/building supply companies

EcoClean
2828 N. 36th St.
Phoenix, AZ 85008
602-224-5313
www.ecoclean-az.com
www.thehealthyhomesolution.com

EcoClean is your asthma and allergy store. They create clean rooms and detoxify homes for healthy life styles and the chemically sensitive. How: Organic mattresses and bedding, air purification systems, organic and zero VOC paints, natural flooring, and organic floor cleaning services.

Allergy Buyers Club
Boston Green Goods, Inc.
45 Braintree Hill Park, Suite 300
Braintree, MA 02184
781-419-5500
www.allergybuyersclub.com

Allergy Buyers Club is your source for furniture, filters, beddings, cleaners and more. Since 1999, they have been an authorized online retailer by numerous manufacturers for all of the healthy home products they sell and a trusted source for honest product reviews and ratings. The company is also a top rated member of the Better Business Bureau.

Ecohaus
819 Southeast Taylor Street
Portland, OR 97214
503-222-3881
www.ecohaus.com

Ecohaus produces environmentally friendly building supplies. At ecohaus, they believe that everyone cares about the health of the planet. Not just movie stars, activists and dreamers, but every one of us. We all want to live in a world with clean air, abundant forests, thriving communities and a future full of promise.

At the same time, they realize that anyone who builds or remodels has one priority above all: to create a beautiful, healthy home where everything works.

Ecohaus connects these two ideals simply by offering the best building products made locally and around the world.

ARTEMIS

3709 Butler Street
Pittsburgh, PA 15201
877-297-8267
www.artemisenvironmental.com

ARTEMIS Environmental Building Materials displays and sells high-quality, environmentally responsible, "green" building products. Opened in Pittsburgh in the spring of 2005, ARTEMIS is designed to expand the availability and use of green building products in the tri-state region.

The products that you'll find at ARTEMIS were selected because they are better for the environment, perform well, and contribute to healthier living. You'll be able to see, touch, smell and purchase materials you may have read about but were not previously accessible. You'll find new options for improving your home or business environment.

Green Depot
Numerous store locations
212-226-0444 - Orders
877-883-4733 - Build Desk
www.greendepot.com
email: contactus@greendepot.com

Green Depot is a resource for the kitchen and home, paints, furniture, filters, and more.

Green Depot is a leading supplier of environmentally friendly and sustainable building products, services and home solutions. The primary goal is to facilitate green living and building in communities so that it is easy, affordable and gratifying.

Founded in 2005 by Sarah Beatty, Green Depot's mission has been - from the outset - to make green building products and services readily accessible so that green building can be easily adopted into standard construction operations. Their goal has been to help establish sustainable building as cost competitive, and provide products of the highest quality that are certified green.

Dietary Supplements

Health Freedom Nutrition
255 Bell Street
Reno, NV 89503
800-980-8780
www.hfn-usa.com

Health Freedom Nutrition is known throughout the industry as a producer of Advanced Nutritional Formulations. Dr. Marianne Marchese chose Health Freedom Nutrition to manufacture and distribute her Estro Relief™, Hepa Cleanse™ and Detox Cofactors™ products mentioned in this book.

Cosmetics and Beauty

Campaign for Safe Cosmetics

www.safecosmetics.org

The Campaign for Safe Cosmetics is a coalition effort launched in 2004 to protect the health of consumers and workers by securing the corporate, regulatory and legislative reforms necessary to eliminate dangerous chemicals from cosmetics and personal care products.

Skin Deep

1436 U Street. NW, Suite 100
Washington, DC 20009
202-667-6982
www.cosmeticdatabase.com

Skin Deep is a safety guide to cosmetics and personal care products brought to you by researchers at the Environmental Working Group. You are able to search for a product, ingredient or company on this site.

Organic Consumers Association

www.organicconsumers.org/bodycare

The Organic Consumers Association (OCA) is an online and grassroots non-profit 501(c)(3) public interest organization campaigning for health, justice, and sustainability. The OCA deals with crucial issues of food safety, industrial agriculture, genetic engineering, children's health, and corporate accountability. They list brands that market their products as "organic," but they don't have enough organic ingredients to be USDA certified, and they use ingredients that would never be allowed in USDA certified products.

Colon Hydrotherapy

Prime Pacific Health Innovations
800-223-9374
www.thecolonet.com

Prime Pacific Health Innovations Corporation (PPHIC) was established in 1997 with the mission to be the world leader in the field of colon hydrotherapy.

Clearwater Colon Hydrotherapy, Inc
3145 S.W. 74th Terrace
Ocala, FL 34474-6498
352-401-0303
www.colonhydrotherapy.com

Mary Ruth Baker has been in the field of colon hydrotherapy for over 30 years. Her commitment has always been to have the highest standard of quality and client care. These high standards are now available in Clearwater Colon Hydrotherapy Systems. These systems have the best mechanical and operational design. Mary Ruth feels that Clearwater Colon Hydrotherapy has created the ultimate in colon hydrotherapy equipment.

Sauna Companies

Heavenly Heat Saunas
PO Box 2892
Crested Butte, CO 81224
970-349-6846; 800-697-2862 (1-800 My Sauna)
www.heavenlyheatsaunas.com
email: Info@HeavenlyHeatSaunas.com

Heavenly Heat Saunas have built the highest quality "chemically-safest" saunas for environmentally ill persons for 22 years. Saunas that are safest for chemically sensitive persons are naturally ideal for anyone's detoxification needs. All types of saunas are available: Finnish (the traditional type), Far-infrared, and combination models with both heating systems. Near-infrared heating can also be included. Each sauna is hand built to-order in the USA.

SaunaRay
P.O. Box 188, Collingwood,
Ontario, Canada L9Y 3Z5
1-877-992-1100
www.saunaray.com
email: info@saunaray.com

SaunaRay is a North American manufacturer of medical grade infrared saunas. All units are ergonomically designed with the comfort of the user in mind. They can be placed on any floor surface, require no drains or vents, and can be moved in a minivan. SaunaRay builds the industry's only "medical grade" saunas which are completely free of toxin building material and come with a built-in Lifetime Guarantee.

Advanced Training for Physicians

Teleosis Institute
863 Arlington Ave.
Berkeley, CA 94707
Phone: 510-558-7285
www.teleosis.org
email: info@teleosis.org

The Teleosis Institute is devoted to developing effective, sustainable health care provided by professionals who serve as environmental health stewards.

Teleosis is dedicated to reducing healthcare's footprint while broadening its ecological vision. They believe in a health care system that conserves natural resources, promotes personal wellness, and begins with precaution. At the forefront of this sustainable medical system are health providers who take an active role in greening healthcare through example, education and advocacy.

American College for the Advancement of Medicine
8001 Irvine Center Drive, Suite 825
Irvine, CA 92618
1-800-532-3688
www.acam.org

The American College for Advancement in Medicine (ACAM) is a not-for-profit corporation dedicated to educating physicians and other health care professionals on the latest findings and emerging procedures in complementary, alternative and integrative (CAIM) medicine. ACAM's healthcare model focuses on prevention of illness and a strive for total wellness. ACAM is the voice of integrative medicine; their goals are to improve physician skills, knowledge and diagnostic procedures as they relate to integrative medicine; to support integrative medicine research; and to provide education on current standard of care as well as additional approaches to patient care.

Spiritmed
17028 E El Pueblo Blvd
Fountain Hills, AZ 85268
www.crinnionmedical.com

This post-graduate training in environmental medicine is provided by Dr. Walter Crinnion. It is a certification Course on Environmental Medicine for Healthcare Professionals that Dr. Marianne Marchese took in 2003.

In 2011, they have joined forces with the American College for Advancement in Medicine (ACAM) to provide training in Environmental Medicine.

Institute of Women's Health and Integrative Medicine
www.instituteofwomenshealth.com

The Institute of Women's Health and Integrative Medicine offers post-graduate training in women's health provided by Dr. Tori Hudson. The institute is an educational and research organization whose mission is to provide advanced training to primary health care practitioners and to conduct and support clinical research in women's health and natural therapies and integrative medicine.

The institute offers quarterly seminars that, in total, constitute a unique 2-year curriculum. The seminars cover menstrual disorders, menopause (offered once yearly), pelvic tumors/ pelvic pain/ urogynecology, women's cancers, primary care for women, STIs/ contraception, and special topics.

Dr. Marianne Marchese feels this is the best continuing education for a physician that exists in the US.

Labs for Environmental Testing

Doctor's Data Lab
3755 Illinois Ave.
St. Charles, IL 60174
800-323-2784 (US & Canada) 630-377-8139 (Elsewhere)
www.doctorsdata.com
email: inquiries@doctorsdata.com

Doctor's Data, Inc. (DDI), a premier clinical laboratory with over 35 years' experience, provides specialty testing to healthcare practitioners around the world.

A specialist and pioneer in essential and toxic elemental testing of multiple human tissues, the laboratory offers a wide array of functional testing. DDI's tests are utilized in the assessment, detection, prevention, and treatment of heavy metal burden, nutritional deficiencies, gastrointestinal function, hepatic detoxification, metabolic abnormalities, and diseases of environmental origin.

They are the leader in heavy metal testing and offer home water testing kits for the public.

Great Plains Lab
11813 West 77th Street
Lenexa, KS 66214 USA
Toll Free (USA, Canada, and Puerto Rico): 800-288-0383
Local: 913-341-8949
www.greatplainslaboratory.com
e-mail: CustomerService@GPL4U.com

The Great Plains Laboratory, Inc. is the world leader in providing testing for nutritional factors in chronic illnesses such as fibromyalgia, autism and ADD.

They offer a variety of metabolic tests such as immune deficiency evaluation, amino acid tests, essential fatty acid tests, glutathione levels, metal toxicity and food allergies tests.

Metametrix
3425 Corporate Way
Duluth, GA 30096 USA
800-221-4640
www.metametrix.com

Much of the healthcare industry is focused on treating symptoms rather than investigating underlying causes of disease. At Metametrix, their mission is to improve health worldwide by providing clinical laboratory services in the area of nutrients, toxicants, hormonal balance, biotransformation and detoxification, and gastrointestinal function. They provide testing for heavy metals, solvents, pesticides and other chemicals.

US BioTek Laboratories
13500 Linden Ave North
Seattle, WA 98133
877-318-8728 (US or Canada)
www.usbiotek.com

US BioTek Laboratories strives to be a leader and innovator in cutting edge laboratory medicine. Our goal is to provide our clients with reliable, quality service through state-of-the-art technology and continuous research.

The commitment, dedication, and integrity of our exceptional team of employees ensure not only the success of our company, but that we will make a qualitative difference in the healthcare industry.

They offer a simple urine solvent test that also checks for phthalates and parabens.

Genova Diagnostics
63 Zillicoa Street
Asheville, NC 28801
800-522-4762
www.genovadiagnostics.com

Genova Diagnostics is a global leader in functional laboratory testing, pioneering innovative new approaches to personalized medicine.

Patients and clinicians focusing on wellness and prevention and taking an active role in managing health prefer diagnostic tests designed to help identify problems before chronic conditions and diseases develop. Unlike traditional labs that focus on disease pathology, Genova specializes in comprehensive panels that combine standard and innovative biomarkers to provide a more complete understanding of specific biological systems.

They offer testing for single nucleotide polymorphisms, SNPs.

Water Testing

Doctor's Data Lab
3755 Illinois Ave.
St. Charles, IL 60174
800-323-2784 (US & Canada) 630-377-8139 (Elsewhere)
www.doctorsdata.com
email: inquiries@doctorsdata.com

See details under "Labs for Environmental Testing." They offer home water testing.

National Testing Laboratories
6571 Wilson Mills Rd.
Cleveland, OH 44143
800-458-3330 or 440-449-2525
www.ntllabs.com
www.watercheck.com
e-mail: ntlsales@ntllabs.com

The National Testing Laboratories, Ltd. Network (NTL) is one of the largest independent laboratories in the U.S. specializing in drinking water analysis for compliance and information. The network laboratories successfully participate in USEPA Proficiency Testing Programs and hold multiple certifications across the U.S.

Test packages are offered to meet state, FDA and International Bottled Water Association requirements. NTL's technical staff is contributing members of various IBWA committees.

Center for Environmental Quality at Wilkes University
Water Research Center
B.F. Environmental Consultants Inc.
15 Hillcrest Drive
Dallas, PA 18612
www.water-research.net
email: bfenviro@ptd.net

Website dedicated to information for private well owners, evaluation of water and wastewater treatment systems, and education/outreach programs. They offer home water testing.

GLOSSARY
THE CULPRITS

The following list is a glossary and comes from referenced sources, The Centers for Disease Control, The U.S. Environmental Protection Agency, and The Agency for Toxic Substances and Disease Registry.

Acetone

Acetone is a chemical that is found naturally in the environment. It is a colorless liquid with a strong odor and taste. It is flammable, and dissolves in water. Acetone is used to make plastic, fibers, drugs, and other chemicals. It is also used to dissolve other substances and is often used in the cosmetic industry. It can be found in plants, trees, volcanic gases, forest fires, and as a byproduct of the breakdown of body fat. It is present in vehicle exhaust, tobacco smoke, nail-polish remover, cleaners and landfill sites. Most know acetone best as the stinky stuff in our nail polish remover. We inhale it and absorb it through our skin. Acetone is not good for your health.

Arsenic

Arsenic is a naturally occurring heavy metal found deep within the earth. In the environment, organic arsenic forms inorganic arsenic compounds, which are mainly used to preserve wood. It is called Copper Chromated Arsenic (CCA) and is used to make "pressure-treated" lumber. It has been used to make wood decks in homes and wood jungle gyms at schools and parks. CCA is no longer used in the U.S. for residential uses; however, it is still used in industrial applications. Organic arsenic compounds are used as pesticides, primarily on cotton plants. Arsenic accumulates in the soil, and food grown in it may contain arsenic. Arsenic is also in the waterways and is present in shellfish. It is a known carcinogen and can cause changes to the skin such as hyperpigmentation and rashes.

Asbestos

Asbestos is really six different fibrous minerals (amosite, chrysotile, crocidolite, and the fibrous varieties of tremolite, actinolite, and anthophyllite) that occur naturally in the environment. Asbestos has been used for a wide range of manufactured goods, mostly in building materials (roofing shingles, ceiling and floor tiles, paper products, and asbestos cement products), friction products (automobile clutches, brakes, and transmission parts), heat-resistant fabrics, packaging, gaskets, and coatings. Also, some vermiculite or talc products may contain asbestos. Asbestos is highly carcinogenic and linked to lung cancer, among other health problems.

Benzene

Benzene is a solvent that is a colorless liquid with a sweet odor. It is highly flammable and occurs both naturally and is man-made. Benzene is widely used in the United States; it ranks in the top 20 chemicals for production volume. It is a main contributor to air pollution as it is produced from auto-exhaust and cigarette smoke. Some industries use benzene to make other chemicals, which are used to make plastics, resins, and nylon and synthetic fibers. Benzene is also used to make some types of rubbers, lubricants, dyes, detergents, drugs, and pesticides. Benzene is also produced from forest fires and volcanoes. Again, air pollution is the main source of daily exposure.

Bisphenol-A (BPA)

Bisphenol-A is found in many products that we come into contact with every day. It is a known environmental estrogen. It is used to manufacture polycarbonate plastic (bottles); it is in the plastic lining of metal food cans; and it is also in dental sealants for composite fillings. Heating can cause BPA to leach as in the sterilization of food cans and washing of polycarbonate plastic bottles. BPA is a contaminant in our drinking and bathing water. It causes hormonal and reproductive problems in humans.[1]

1,3-Butadiene

1,3-Butadiene is a chemical made from the processing of petroleum. About 65% of the manufactured 1,3-butadiene is used to make synthetic rubber used for tires on cars and trucks. It is also used to make plastics including acrylics. Small amounts are also found in gasoline. Exposure is mainly from air pollution.

Cadmium

Cadmium is a naturally occurring heavy metal found deep within the earth. All soils and rocks, including coal and mineral fertilizers, contain some cadmium. Since cadmium is in the soil, it can accumulate in vegetables grown in contaminated soil. Most cadmium used in the United States is extracted during the production of other metals like zinc, lead, and copper. Cadmium has many uses, including batteries, pigments, metal coatings, and plastics. Cadmium is also a contaminant in cigarette smoke and vegetables grown in contaminated soil. It accumulates up the food chain and is found as a contaminant in many foods.

Chloroform

Chloroform is a colorless liquid that will burn when it reaches very high temperatures.

In the past, chloroform was used as an inhaled anesthetic during surgery. Today, chloroform is used to make other chemicals. Also, it can be formed in small amounts when chlorine is added to water by a city to be used as a disinfectant and then that water is heated during bathing or showering. Other names for chloroform are trichloromethane, trihalomethanes (see below) and methyl trichloride. Showering, bathing and drinking unfiltered city water are the main sources of exposure.

DDT

DDT (dichlorodiphenyltrichloroethane) is an organochlorine pesticide once widely used in agriculture and to eradicate insects that carry diseases such as malaria. Its use in the U.S. was banned in 1972 because of damage to wildlife, but it is still used in some countries. Even in the U.S. it is still detected in the soil, lakes and rivers and is found in foods. DDE (dichlorodiphenyldichloroethylene) is a metabolite of DDT. DDE has no commercial use. DDT and DDE have been linked to numerous health conditions in humans, including breast cancer.

Dioxin

Dioxins are not manufactured for any use in any product or food. They are an unwanted byproduct in the production of chlorinated hydrocarbons, pesticides, wood preservatives, paper production, and incineration of plastics. It is a contaminant in the air, soil, rivers and lakes and accumulates up the food chain. Dioxin is a general term for 75 different compounds. The most toxic is known as TCDD, 2,3,7,8-tetrachlorodibenzo-p-dioxin. Dioxins affect the immune system and hormonal system of humans.[2]

Ethylene glycol/Propylene glycol

Both ethylene glycol and propylene glycol are used to make antifreeze and de-icing solutions for cars, airplanes, and boats; to make polyester compounds; and as solvents in the paint and plastics industries. Ethylene glycol is also an ingredient in photographic developing solutions, hydraulic brake fluids and in inks used in stamp pads, ballpoint pens, and print shops. The Food and Drug Administration (FDA) has classified propylene glycol as an additive that is "generally recognized as safe" for use in food. It is used to absorb extra water and maintain moisture in certain medicines, cosmetics, or food products. It is a solvent for food colors and flavors.

Formaldehyde

Formaldehyde is a chemical used widely by various industries to manufacture building materials and numerous household products. It is also a byproduct of combustion and certain other natural processes. It is a volatile organic compound (VOC) used in the production of fertilizer, paper, plywood, and urea-formaldehyde resins. It is also used as a preservative in some foods and in many products used around the house, such as antiseptics, medicines, and cosmetics. It is in cabinets and furniture made from particleboard, plywood, and fiberboard. It is found in foam insulation, cigarette smoke and some clothing. Formaldehyde can cause allergic reactions, hormonal disruption and other adverse health conditions.[3]

Heterocyclic Amines (HCA)

Heterocyclic Amines are chemicals produced from cooking muscle meat at high temperatures. They are formed when amino acids and creatine (from muscle) react at high temperatures. There are over 17 different HCAs that can be formed from cooking fish, beef, pork and chicken and all are carcinogenic.[4]

Lead

Lead is a naturally occurring bluish-gray metal found in small amounts in the earth's crust. Much of it comes from human activities including burning fossil fuels, mining, and manufacturing. It is used in the production of batteries, ammunition, metal products (solder and pipes), and devices to shield X-rays. Because of health concerns, lead from gasoline, paints and ceramic products, caulking, pipe, pesticides, and food containers has been dramatically reduced in recent years but it still remains in the environment. Currently the main sources of exposure are old homes with lead paint, drinking water from leaching of old pipes, ceramics, and food grown in contaminated soil. Most recently, lead has been found in children's toys imported from China. The adverse health effects of lead are well documented.[5]

Mercury

Mercury is a naturally occurring metal that has several forms. Mercury combines with other elements, such as chlorine, sulfur, or oxygen, to form inorganic mercury compounds or "salts," which are usually white powders or crystals. Mercury also combines with carbon to make organic mercury compounds. The most common one, methylmercury, is produced mainly by microscopic organisms in the water and soil. More mercury in the environment can increase the amount of methylmercury that these small organisms make. Metallic mercury is used to produce chlorine gas and caustic soda, and is also used in thermometers, dental fillings, and batteries. Mercury salts are sometimes used in skin-lightening creams and as antiseptic creams and ointments. The FDA has recently released a warning about mercury fillings and dangers to human health. Methylmercury is the most toxic form of mercury and is found in fish.

Organochlorine compounds

Organochlorine compounds are a group of chemical compounds with many uses. They are organic compounds containing at least one chlorine atom. The simplest form is chlorinated hydrocarbons. They include pesticides chloroform, solvents such as trichloroethylene, and polychlorinated biphenols. Some are naturally occurring and some are man-made, like dioxins. They are used in pesticides, such as DDT, aldrin and dieldrin, which had numerous adverse health effects and are no longer used in the U.S.[6]

Organophosphate compounds

Organophosphate compounds are a group of chemical compounds with many uses. They are also the basis of many insecticides, herbicides, and nerve gases, such as parathion, malathion, methyl parathion, chlorpyrifos, and diazinon. Organophosphates are widely used as solvents, and plasticizers.[6]

Parabens

Parabens are antimicrobial agents used in cosmetics, lotions, soaps, shampoos, conditioners, foods and a wide variety of other consumer products. The three forms of commercially used parabens are ethyl-(EP), methyl-(MP), and propyl-(PP) paraben. Parabens are absorbed through the skin and accumulate in the body. They are known allergens and are estrogenic chemicals linked to hormonal conditions in men and women.[7]

Pentachlorophenol

Pentachlorophenol is a manufactured chemical that is a restricted-use pesticide and is used industrially as a wood preservative for utility poles, railroad ties, and wharf pilings. Exposure to high levels of pentachlorophenol can cause increases in body temperature, liver effects, damage to the immune system, reproductive effects, and developmental effects. This substance has been found in at least 313 of the 1,585 National Priorities List sites identified by the Environmental Protection Agency (EPA). Pentachlorophenol can be found in the air, water, and soil. It enters the environment through evaporation from treated wood surfaces, industrial spills, and disposal at uncontrolled hazardous waste sites. Pentachlorophenol is broken down by sunlight, other chemicals, and microorganisms into other chemicals within a couple of days to months. Pentachlorophenol is found in fish and other foods, but tissue levels are usually low. *http://www.atsdr.cdc.gov*

Pesticides

Pesticides are chemical agents used to eradicate some living organism. They include herbicides, insecticides and fungicides. The organochlorine compounds were the first synthetic pesticides to be used and include DDT, aldrin, atrazine, dieldrin, and lindane. They have low water solubility and high chemical stability. They are lipophilic compounds (fat-loving) and bioaccumulate and move up the food chain into wildlife and humans. Most have been banned in the U.S. due to harmful health effects in humans. Organophosphate pesticides have mostly replaced the organochlorines and include methylparathion and ethylparathion, which are used in agriculture to control pests in this country and others. They have adverse health effects on human reproduction.[8] Parathion, malathion, and atropine are also used in agriculture to control mosquitoes, and malathion is used in shampoos and lotions for lice treatment. These have adverse health effects on humans, including links to breast cancer.[9]

Phenol

Phenol is both a manufactured chemical and a natural substance. You can taste and smell phenol at levels lower than those that are associated with harmful effects. Phenol is used primarily in the production of phenolic resins and in the manufacture of nylon and other synthetic fibers. It is also found in wood preservatives. It is also used in slimicides (chemicals that kill bacteria and fungi in slimes), as a disinfectant and antiseptic, and in medicinal preparations such as mouthwash and sore throat lozenges. Phenols are used to make other chemicals such as pentachlorophenol used in wood and pesticides, and has been shown to cause disruption to a woman's hormonal system.[10]

Phthalates

Phthalates are man-made chemicals used in plastics and numerous consumer products. Human exposure is mostly through food and water. They are in polyvinyl chloride (PVC) products including upholstery, tablecloths, shower curtains, children's toys, and raincoats. They are used in pesticides, cosmetics, perfume, nail polish, plastic bottles, and medical supplies such as plastic IV tubing, plastic Tupperware, and many more items. They are considered hormone-disruptors and have known harmful effects to both men and women. These are discussed in depth throughout the book.[11]

Polybrominated diphenyl ether (PBDEs)

Polybrominated Diphenyl ethers are flame-retardant chemicals that are added to a variety of consumer products to make them resistant to fires. Because PBDEs are added to the product, they could leave the product under ideal conditions and enter the environment. They are in electrical devices such as computers and TV sets, furniture and fabric, plastics and foam. They are released over time and inhaled by humans and contaminate food and water. They have been found in the adipose tissue and breast milk of women. They have known adverse health effects.

Polychlorinated Biphenols (PCBs)

Polychlorinated Biphenyls are mixtures of up to 209 individual chlorinated compounds (known as congeners). There are no known natural sources of PCBs.

PCBs have been used as coolants, flame retardants, and lubricants in transformers, capacitors, and other electrical equipment because they don't burn easily and are good insulators. The manufacture of PCBs was stopped in the U.S. in 1977 because of evidence that they build up in the environment and can cause harmful health effects. Products made before 1977 that may contain PCBs include old fluorescent lighting fixtures and electrical devices containing PCB capacitors, and old microscope and hydraulic oils. Because of resistance to degradation, PCBs persist in the environment for decades and have adverse health effects.

Polycyclic Aromatic Hydrocarbons (PAHs)

Polycyclic Aromatic Hydrocarbons (PAHs) are a group of over 100 different chemicals that are formed during the incomplete burning of coal, oil and gas, garbage, or other organic substances like tobacco or charbroiled meat. Some PAHs are manufactured. These pure PAHs usually exist as colorless, white, or pale yellow-green solids. PAHs are found in coal tar, crude oil, creosote, and roofing tar, but a few are used in medicines or to make dyes, plastics, and pesticides. The main source of exposure is food and air pollution. These are known carcinogens.

Platinum
Platinum is a heavy metal that occurs naturally in the earth. It is a silvery-white metal that is malleable and ductile, and resistant to corrosion. The metal does not oxidize in air and is used as a catalyst for many industrial processes. Platinum is used in dentistry, chemotherapeutic agents, jewelry, and silicone breast implants.

Solvents
A solvent is a liquid substance that is capable of dissolving one or more other substances. Solvents are organic chemicals called organic solvents, often referred to as volatile organic compounds (VOCs). Common uses are in dry-cleaning (tetrchloroethylene), paint thinner (toluene), nail polish removers (acetone), plastics and styrofoam (styrene), paints, cigarette smoke and gasoline (xylene, benzene). Many of these are carcinogenic.[12]

Toluene
Toluene is a clear, colorless liquid with a distinctive smell. Toluene occurs naturally in crude oil and in the tolu tree. It is also produced in the process of making gasoline and other fuels from crude oil and making coke from coal. Toluene is used in making paints, paint thinners, fingernail polish, lacquers, adhesives, and rubber and in some printing and leather-tanning processes.[12]

Tetrachloroethylene (TERC)(PERC)
Tetrachloroethylene is a manufactured chemical that is widely used for dry-cleaning of fabrics and for metal-degreasing. It is also used to make other chemicals and is used in some consumer products. Other names for tetrachloroethylene include perchloroethylene, PERC, and tetrachloroethene. When you bring clothes from the dry

cleaners, they will release small amounts of tetrachloroethylene into the air. It also contaminated the water and air. TERC is a known carcinogen and has numerous adverse health effects.

Trichloroethylene (TCE)

Trichloroethylene (TCE) is used mainly as a solvent to remove grease from metal parts, but it is also an ingredient in adhesives, paint removers, typewriter correction fluids, and spot removers. It is also used in the dry-cleaning industry. Trichloroethylene is not thought to occur naturally in the environment. It is mostly a byproduct from manufacturing and ends up in the water, air and soil due to industrial contamination. It has been found in underground water sources and many surface waters as a result of contamination. The main source of exposure is air and water. It has mostly been replaced by tetrachloroethylene, which is used in dry-cleaning.[12]

Trihalomethanes

Trihalomethanes are a group of four chemicals that are formed along with other disinfection byproducts when chlorine or other disinfectants used to control microbial contaminants in drinking water react with naturally occurring organic and inorganic matter in water. The trihalomethanes are chloroform (see above), bromodichloromethane, dibromochloromethane, and bromoform. They can form during showering or bathing. The main source of exposure is through the air and contact with water or drinking water with high levels. These are known carcinogens and have other adverse health effects.

Volatile organic compounds (VOCs)

Volatile organic compounds (VOCs) are emitted as gases from certain solids or liquids. VOCs can include chemicals, which may have short- and long-term adverse health effects. Concentrations of many VOCs are higher indoors than outdoors. VOCs are emitted by a wide array of products, including; paints and lacquers, paint strippers, cleaning supplies, pesticides, building materials and furnishings, office equipment such as copiers and printers, correction fluids, permanent markers, and photographic solutions. They are found in household products, paints, varnishes, and cleaning, disinfecting, cosmetic, degreasing, and hobby products.[12]

References

Introduction

1. Bergstrom R, et al. *J Natl Cancer Inst.* 1996;88(11):727-733.
2. Rea WJ. *Chemical Sensitivity Vol 1,2,3.* Boca Raton, FL: Lewis Publ;1992, 1994, 1996.
3. Welshons WV, et al. Large effects from small exposures. Mechanism for endocrine-disrupting chemicals with estrogenic activity. *Environ Health Perspect.* 2003;111:994-1006.
4. Crinnion WJ. Environmental medicine, part 1: The human burden of environmental toxins and their common health effects. *Altern Med Rev* 2000;5(1):52-63.

Chapter I

1. Nicolopoulou-Stamati P, Pitsos MA. The impact of endocrine disruptors on the female reproductive system. *Human Repr Update* 2001;7(3):323-330.
2. Rajapakse N, Silva E, Kortenkamp A. Combining xenoestrogens at low levels below individual no-observed-effect concentrations dramatically enhances steroid hormone action. *Environ Health Perspect.* 2002;110(9):917-21.
3. www.ewg.org/sites/humantoxome/ and www.ewg.org/featured/15.
4. www.cdc.gov/exposurereport.
5. www.pollutioninpeople.org.
6. www.calbbc.org.
7. www.pbs.org/tradesecrets/problem/bodyburden.

Chapter II

Food

1. www.ewg.org.
2. Gunderson EL. FDA total diet study, July 1986-April 1991, dietary intakes of pesticides, selected elements, and other chemicals. JAOAC Int 1995;78(6):1353-1363.
3. Levin, B. *Environmental Nutrition.* Hingepin Publ Vashon Island, WA 1999;151-164.
4. Wolfe MF, Seiber JN. Environmental activation of pesticides. *Occupational Med* 1993;8(3):561-573.
5. Clarkson TW. The three modern faces of mercury. *Environ Health Perspec.* 2002;110(1):11-23.
6. http://www.usatoday.com/news/health/2007-10-29-mercury-cover_N.htm.
7. Serrano R, Blanes MA, lopez FJ. Biomagnifications of organochlorine pollutants in farmed and wild gilthead sea bream and stable isotope characterization of the tropic chains. *Sci Total Environ.* 2008;389(2-3):340-349.
8. Shaw SD, et al. PCBs, PCDD/Fs, and organochlorine pesticides in farmed Atlantic salmon from Maine, eastern Canada, and Norway, and wild salmon from Alaska. *Environ Sci Technol.* 2006;40(17):5347-5354.
9. Vom Saal FS, Hughes C. An extensive new literature concerning low-dose effects of bisphenol-A shows the need for new risk assessment. *Environ health Perspect.* 2005;113(8);926-933.
10. Lang IA, et al. Association of urinary bisphenol-A concentration with medical disorders and laboratory abnormalities in adults. JAMA. 2008 ;300 :1303-1310.
11. Levin, B. *Environmental Nutrition.* Hingepin Publ. Vashon Island, WA. 1999 Chapter 4.

12. Tsumura Y, et al. Eleven phthalate esters and di(2-ethylhexyl) adipate in one-week duplicate diet sample obtained from hospitals and their estimated daily intake. *Food Addit Contam.* 2001;18(5):4490460.

13. Jouni JK, et al. The role of exposure to phthalates from polyvinyl chloride products in the development of asthma and allergies: A systematic review and meta-analysis. *Environ Health Perspect.* 2008;116:845-853.

14. Levin, B. *Environmental Nutrition.* Hingepin Publ. Vashon Island, WA. 1999 Chapter 3,4.

15. Moore, G. *Living with the Earth:Concepts in Environmental Medicine.* 2ed Lewis Publishers. Boca Raton, FL. 2002 Chapter 5.

Water

1. Moore, G. *Living with the Earth: Concepts in Environmental Medicine.* 2ed Lewis Publishers. Boca Raton, FL. 2002 Chapter 9.

2. Whitaker HJ, Nieuwenhuijsen MJ, Best NG. The relationship between water concentrations and individual uptake of chloroform: A simulation study. *Environ Health Perspect.* 2003:111(5);688-694.

3. Jaakkola Jouni JK, knight, T. The role of exposure to phthalates from polyvinyl chloride products in the development of asthma and allergies: A systematic review and meta-analysis. *Environ Health Perspect* 2008:116;845-853.

4. Lovenkamp-Swan, T, Davis, BJ. Mechanisms of phthalate ester toxicity in the female reproductive system. *Environ Health Perspect* 2003:111(2);139-145.

5. Vom Saal, FS, Hughes, C. An extensive new literature concerning low-dose effects pf Bisphenol-A shows the need for new risk assessment. *Environ Health Perspect* 2005;113(8);926-933.

6. Tobias, L. Graduate from plastic. *Natural Home Magazine.* 2003 May/June.78-80.

Air

1. Kunzli N, Tager IB. Long-term health effects of particulate and other ambient air pollution: Research can progress faster if we want it to. *Environ Health Perspect.* 2000:108(10);915-918.
2. www.epa.gov/air.
3. Cohen AJ. Outdoor Air Pollution and Lung Cancer. *Environ Health Perspect* 2000:108(supp4);743-750.
4. A healthy home environment. *Environ Health Perspect* 1999;107(7);1-7.

Products and Cosmetics

1. Zhang Y, et al. Hair-coloring product use and risk of non-hodgkin's lymphoma: a population-based case-control study in Connecticut. *Am J Epidemiol.* 2004;159(2):148-154.
2. Zahm SH, et al. Use of hair coloring products and the risk of lymphoma, multiple myeloma, and chronic lymphocytic leukemia. *Am J Public Health.* 1993;82(4):598-599.
3. Duty S, et al. Personal care product use predicts urinary concentrations of some phthalate monoesters. *Environ health Perspect.* 2005;113:1530-1535.
4. Eisenhardt S, et al. Nitromusk compounds in women with gynecological and endocrine dysfunction. *Environ Res Sec A* 2001;87:123-130.
5. Natural solutions magazine. 2010;Jan/Feb:29-31.

Chapter Three

Breast Cancer

1. *State of the Evidence 2008: The Connection Between Breast Cancer and the Environment,* edited by Janet Gray, Ph.D., and published by the Breast Cancer Fund. www.breastcancerfund. org.
2. Aschengrau et al, Occupational exposure to estrogenic chemicals and the occurrence of breast cancer: an exploratory analysis *AM J Ind Med.* 1998 ;34(1) :6-14.

3. Welshons WV, et al. Large effects from small exposures. I. Mechanisms for endocrine-disrupting chemicals with estrogenic activity. *Environ Health Perspect.* 2003;111:94-1006.

4. Anderson LM, et al. Critical windows of exposure for children's health: cancer in human epidemiological studies and neoplasms in experimental animal models. *Environ Health Perspect.* 2000;108(3):573-594.

5. Cohen BA, et al. DDT and breast cancer in young women: new data on the significance of age at exposure. *Environ Health Perspect.* 2007;115(10):1406-1414.

6. Hirvonen SP, et al. NAT2 slow acetylator genotype as an important modifier of breast cancer risk. *Int J Cancer.* 2005;114(4):579-584.

7. Coutille C, et al. Risk factors in alcohol associated breast cancer: alcohol dehydrogenase polymorphisms and estrogens. *Int J oncol* 2004;25(4):1127-1132.

8. Seitz HK, becker P. Alcohol metabolism and cancer risk. *Alcohol Res Health.* 2007;30(1):38-41.

9. Brody JG, et al. Environmental pollutants and breast cancer:epidemiolic studies. *Cancer.* 2007;109:2667-2711.

10. Gammon MD, et al. Environmental toxins and breast cancer on Long Island. I. Polycyclic aromatic hydrocarbon DNA adducts. *Cancer Epidemiol Biomarkers Prev.* 2002 Aug;11(8):677-85.

11. Warner MB, et al. Serum dioxin concentrations and breast cancer risk in the Seveso women's health study. *Environ Health Perspect.* 2002;110(625-628.

12. Welshons WV, Nagel SC, Vom Saal FS. Large effects from small exposures III: Endocrine mechanisms mediating effects of bisphenol A at levels of human exposure. *Endocrinology.* 2006;147:S56-S69.

13. Cohen BA, et al. DDT and breast cancer in young women: New data on the significance of age at exposure. *Environ Health Perspect.* 2007;115:1406-1414.

14. Dewailly E, et al. High organochlorine body burden in women with estrogen receptor positive breast cancer. *J of Natl Cancer Inst*. 1994;86(3):232-234.

15. Teitelbaum SL, et al. Reported residential pesticide use and breast cancer risk on long island, NY. *AM J Epidemiol*. 2006;165:643-651.

16. Debruin LS, Josephy PD. Perspectives on the chemical etiology of breast cancer. *Environ Health Perspect*. 2002;110(1):119-127.

17. Lovenkamp-Swan T, Davis BJ. Mechanisms of phthalate ester toxicity in the female reproductive system. *Environ Health Perspect*. 2003;111(2):139-145.

18. Colon I, et al. Identification of phthalate esters in the serum of young Puerto Rican girls with premature breast development. *Environ Health Perspect*. 2000;108:895-900.

19. Kim IY, Han SY, Moon A. Phthalates inhibit tamoxifen-induced apoptosis in MCF-7 human breast cancer cells. *J Toxicol Environ Health*. 2004;67:2025-2035.

20. Darbre PD, et al. Concentrations of parabens in human breast tumors. *J Appl Toxicol*. 2004;24(1):5-13.

21. Byford JR, et al. oestrogenic activity of parabens in MCF7 human breast cancer cells. *J Steroid Biochem*. 2002;80:49-60.

22. Johnson MD, et al. cadmium mimics the in vivo effects of estrogen in the uterus and mammary gland. *Nature Medicine* 2003;9(8):1081-1084.

23. Martin MB, et al. estrogen like activity of metals in MCF7 breast cancer cells. Endocinology. 2003;144:2425-2436.

24. Ionescu JG, et al. Increased levels of transient metals in breast cancer tissue. *Neuroendocinology Letters*. 2006;27(s):36-39.

Endometriosis

1. Frackiewicz E.J. Endometriosis: An overview of the disease and its treatment. *JAM Pharm Assoc* 2000;40(5):645-657.

2. Spaczynski RZ, Duleba AJ. Diagnosis of endometriosis. *Semin Repro Med* 2003;21(2):193-207.

3. 3. Prentice, A. Endometriosis; regular review. *BMJ* 2001;July14;323(7304):93-95.

4. Hellier JF, et al. Organochlorines and endometriosis. *Chemosphere* 2008;71(2):203-210.

5. Cobellis L, et al. High plasma concentrations of di-(2-ethylhexyl)-phthalate in women with endometriosis. *Hum Reprod* 2003;18(7):1512-1515.

6. Reddy BS, et al. Association of phthalate esters with endometriosis in Indian women. *BJOG* 2006;113(5):515-520.

7. Cobellis L, et al. Measurement of bisphenol A and bisphenol B levels in human blood sera from health and endometriotic women. Biomed Chromatogr. 2009 May 14.

8. Foster WG, Agarwal SK. Environmental contaminants and dietary factors in endometriosis. *Ann N Y Acad Sci.* 2002;955:213-29.

9. Taskinen HK, et al. Reduced fertility among female wood workers exposed to formaldehyde. *AM J Indus Med.* 1999;36:206-212.

10. Jackson LW, Zullo MD, Goldberg JM. The association between heavy metals, endometriosis and uterine myomas among premenopausal women: National Health and Nutrition Examination Survey 1999-2002. *Hum Reprod* 2008;23(3):679-687.

11. Hadfield RM, et al. Linkage and association studies of the relationship between endometriosis and genes encoding the detoxification enzymes GSTM1, GSTT1, and CYP1A1. *Mol Hum Reprod* 2001;7(11):1073-1078.

Fibroids of the Uterus

1. Bakas p, et al. Estrogen receptor alpha and beta in uterine fibroids: a basis for altered estrogen responsiveness. *Fertility & Sterility.* 2008;90:1878-1885.

2. Flake GP, Andersen J, Dixon D. Etiology and pathogenesis of uterine leiomyomas: A review. *Environ Health Perspect.* 2002;1111:1037-1054.

3. Gerhard I, et al. Chlorinated hydrocarbons in infertile women. *Env res sec A* 1999;80:299-310.

4. Hunter DS, et al. Influence of exogenous estrogen receptor ligands on uterine leiomyoma: Evidence from an in vitro/in vivo animal model for uterine fibroids. *Environ Health Perspect* 2000;108(S5):829-823.

5. Eskenuzi B, et al. Serum dioxin concentrations and risk of uterine leiomyoma in the Seveso women's health study. *AM J Epidemiol* 2007;166:79-87.

6. Weuve J, Wise L, Hauser r. Association of urinary phthalate concentrations with endometriosis and uterine leiomyomata: Preliminary findings from NHANES 1999-2002. *Epidemiology* 2007;18(5):178-179.

7. Gerhard I, et al. Heavy metals and fertility. *J Toxicol Environ Health Part A* 1998;54:593-611.

8. Jackson LW, Zullo MD, Goldberg JM. The association between heavy metals, endometriosis and uterine myomas among premenopausal women: National Health and Nutrition Examination Survey 1999-2002. *Hum Reprod* 2008;23(3):679-687.

Fibromyalgia, Chronic Fatigue and MCS

1. Sendur OF, et al. The relationship between serum trace element levels and clinical parameters in patients with fibromyalgia. *Rheumatol Int.* 2008;28(11):1117-1121.

2. Engel CC, Adkins JA, Cowen DN. Caring for medically unexplained physical symptoms after toxic environmental exposures: effects of contested causation. *Environ Health Perspect.* 2002;110(4):641-647.

3. Bell IR, et al. Illness from low levels of environmental chemicals: relevance to chronic fatigue syndrome and fibromyalgia. *Am J Med.* 1998;105(3A):74S-82S.

4. Dunstan H, et al. Bioaccumulated chlorinated hydrocarbons and red/white blood cell parameters. *Biochem Mol Med* 1996;58:77-84.

5. Ziem G, McTammey J. Profile of patients with chemical injury and sensitivity. *Environ Health Perspect.* 1997;10(2):417-436.

Heart Disease

1. Ramos K, et al. Responses of vascular smooth muscle cells to toxic insult: Cellular and molecular perspectives for environmental toxicants. *J Toxicol Environ Heath* 1994;43:419-440.

2. Telisman S. et al. Blood Pressure in relation to biomarkers of lead, cadmium, copper, zinc, and selenium in men without occupational exposure to metals. *Environ Res Sec A* 87 2001;87:57-68.

3. Nash D, et al. Blood lead, blood pressure, and hypertension in perimenopausal and postmenopausal women. *JAMA* 2003;289(12):1523-1532.

4. Chan HM, Egeland, GM. Fish consumption, mercury exposure, and heart diseases. *Nutrition Reviews* 2004;62:68-72.

5. Navas-Acien A, et al. Arsenic Exposure and Cardiovascular Disease: A Systematic Review of the Epidemiologic Evidence. *Am J Epid* 2005;162(11):1037-1049.

6. Lang I, et al. Associations of urinary bisphenol A concentrations with medical disorders and laboratory abnormalities in adults. *JAMA* 2008;300(11):1303-1310.

7. Fine LJ. Occupational heart disease. In: Romm WN. *Environmental and Occupational Medicine.* 2nd ed. Boston: Little Brown & Co 1992:593-600.

8. Brook RD. Is air pollution a cause of cardiovascular disease? Updated review and controversies. *Rev Environ Health* 2007;2:115-137.

9. Dubowsky SD, et al. Diabetes, obesity, and hypertension may enhance associations between air pollution and markers of systemic inflammation. *Envion Health Perspect* 2006;114(7):992-998

Infertility
1. http://www.mayoclinic.com
2. Hruska KS, et al. Environmental factors in infertility. *Clinical Obstet Gynecol.* 2000;43(4):821-829.
3. Nicolopoulou-Stamatl P, Pitsos MA. The impact of endocrine disruptors on the female reproductive system. *Hum Reprod Update.* 2001;7(3):323-330.
4. Sharara FI, Seifer DB, Flaws JA. Environmental toxicants and female reproduction. *Fertil Steril.* 1998;70(4):613-622
5. Gerhard I, et al. Chlorinated hydrocarbons in infertile women. *Environ Res Sec A.* 1999;80:200-310.
6. Fei C, et al. Maternal levels of perfluorinated chemicals and subfecundity. *Hum Reprod.* 2009;1(1):1-6
7. Choy CMY, et al. Infertility, blood mercury concentrations and dietary seafood consumption: a case-control study. *BJOG* 2002:109:1121-1125.
8. Patisaul HB, Adewale HB. Long term effects of environmental endocrine disruptors on reproductive physiology and behavior. *Front Behav Neurosci.* 2009;3(10):1-18.
9. Philliips KP, Tanphaichitr N. Human exposure to endocrine disrupters and semen quality. *J Toxicol Environ Health B Crit Rev.* 2008;11(3-4):188-220
10. Latini G, et al. Phthalates exposure and male infertility. *Toxicology.* 2006;226(2-3):90-98

Miscarriage and Premature Birth
1. Hruska KS, et al. Environmental factors in infertility. *Clin Obst Gyn.* 2000;43(4):821-829.
2. Hertz-Picciotto I. The evidence that lead increases the risk for spontaneous abortion. *Am J Ind Med.* 2000;38:300-309.

3. Borja-Aburto V.H, et al. Blood lead levels measured prospectively and risk of spontaneous abortion. *Am J Epid.* 1999;150(6):590-597.
4. Gerhard I, et al. Impact of heavy metal on hormonal and immunological factors in women with repeated miscarriages. *Hum Rep Update.* 1998;4(3):301-309.
5. Sharara Fi, et al. Environmental toxicants and female reproduction. *Fertility and Sterility.* 1998;70(4):613-622.
6. Gerhard I, et al. Chlorinated hydrocarbons in women with repeated miscarriages. *Environ Health Perspect.* 1998;106(10):675-681
7. Nicolopoulou-Stamati P, Pitsos MA. The impact of endocrine disruptors on the female reproductive system. *Hum Rep Update.* 2001;7(3):323-330.
8. Sugiura-Ogasawara M, et al. Exposure to bisphenol A is associated with recurrent miscarriage. *Hum Reprod.* 2005;June 9 advanced access:1-5.
9. Xue F, et al. Maternal fish consumption, mercury levels and risk of preterm delivery. *Environ Health Perspect.* 2007;115(1):42-47
10. Meeker J, et al. Urinary phthalate metabolites in relation to preterm birth in Mexico City. *Environ Health Perspect.* 2008;online June 16:1-30

Osteoporosis

1. Satarug S, Moore M. Adverse health effects of chronic exposure to low-level cadmium in foodstuffs and cigarette smoke. *Environ Health Perspect.* 2004:112:1099-1103.
2. Steassen JA, et al. Environmental exposure to cadmium, forearm bone density, and risk of fractures: prospective population study. *Lancet.* 1999;353:1140-1144.
3. Alfven T, et al. Low-level cadmium exposure and osteoporosis. *J Bone Miner Res.* 2000;15:1579-1586.

4.   Schutte r, et al. Bone resorption and environmental exposure to cadmium in women: A population study. *Environ Health Perspect.* 2008;116(6):777-783.

5.   Potula V, Kaye W. Is lead exposure a risk factor for bone loss? *J Women's Health.* 2005;14(6):461-464.

6.   Vig EK, Hu H. Lead toxicity in older adults. *J Am Geriatr Soc.* 2000:48:1501-1506.

7.   Suzuki Y, et al. Preventive effect of zinc against cadmium-induced bone resorption. *Toxicology.* 1990;62:27-34.

8.   Pande M, et al. Combined administration of a chelating agent and an antioxidant in the prevention and treatment of acute lead intoxication in rats. *Environ Toxicol Pharm.* 2001;9:173-184.

9.   Crinnion WJ. Environmental medicine, part three: long-term effects of chronic low-dose mercury exposure. *Altern Med Rev.* 2000;5(3):209-223.

10. Marini H, et al. Effects of the Phytoestrogen Genistein on Bone Metabolism in Osteopenic Postmenopausal Women. *Ann Intern Med.* 2007;146(12):839-847.

Polycystic Ovarian Syndrome PCOS

1.   Korhonen S, et al. The androgenic sex hormone profile is an essential feature of metabolic syndrome in premenopausal women: a controlled community-based study. *Fertil Steril* 2003;79:1327-1334.

2.   Carmina E. Diagnosing PCOS in women who menstruate regularly. *Contemp OB/GYN* 2003;7:53-63.

3.   De Leo V, Marca AL, Petraglia F. insulin-lowering agents in the management of polycystic ovarian syndrome. *Endocrine Rev* 2003;24(5)633-667.

4.   Alonso-Magdalena P, et al. The estrogenic effect of bisphenol A disrupts pancreatic B-cell function in vivo and induces insulin resistance. *Environ Health Perspect.* 2006;114(1):106-112.

5. Takeuchi T, et al. Positive relationship between androgen and the endocrine disruptor, bisphenol A, in normal women and women with ovarian dysfunction. *Endocrine Journal* 2004:51:165-169.

6. Tsutsumi O. Assessment of human contamination of estrogenic endocrine-disrupting chemicals and their risk for human reproduction. *J Steriod Biochem Mol Biol.* 2005;93:325-330.

7. Lovenkamp-Swan T, Davis BJ. Mechanism of phthalate ester toxicity in the female reproductive system. *Environ Health Perspect.* 2003;111(2):139-145.

8. Davis BJ, Maronpot RR, Heindel JJ. Di-(2-ethylhexyl) phthalate suppresses estradiol and ovulation in cycling rats. *Toxicol Appl Pharmacol.* 1994;128:216-223.

9. Stahlhut RW, et al. Concentrations of urinary phthalate metabolites are associated with increased waist circumference and insulin resistance in adult US males. *Environ Health Perspect.* 2007;115(6):876-882.

10. Gerhard I, et al. Heavy metals and fertility. *J Toxicol Environ Health.* 1998;54:5593-611.

11. Ghanaati Z, et al. Endocrinological and genetic studies in patients with polycystic ovarian syndrome (PCOS). *Neuro Endocrinol Lett.* 1999;20(5):323-327.

Thyroid Disease

1. Kelly G. Peripheral metabolism of thyroid hormones: A review. *Altern Med Rev.* 2000;5(4):306-319.

2. Tomer Y, Huber A. The etiology of autoimmune thyroid disease: a story of genes and environment. *J Autoimmun.* 2009;32(3-4):231-239.

3. www.mayoclinic.com.

4. Brouwer A, et al. Interactions of persistent environmental organochlorines with the thyroid hormone system: Mechanism and possible consequences for animal and human health. *Toxicol Ind Health.* 1998;14:59-84.

5. Scantz SL, Widholm JL. Cognitive effects of endocrine-disrupting chemicals in animals. *Environ Health Perspect.* 2001;109(12):1197-1206.

6. Langer P, et al. Possible effects of polychlorinated biphenyls and organochlorinated pesticides on the thyroid after long-term exposure to heavy environmental pollution. *J Occup Environ Med.* 2003;45:526-532.

7. Koopman-Esseboom C, et al. Effects of dioxins and polychlorinated biphenyls on thyroid hormone status of pregnant women and their infants. *Pediatr Res.* 1994;36:468-473.

8. Panganiban L, et al. Correlation between blood ethylenethiourea and thyroid gland disorders among banana plantation workers in the Philippines. *Environ Health Perspect.* 2004;112(1):42-45.

9. Gerhard I, et al. Pentachlorophenol exposure in women with gynecological and endocrine dysfunction. *Environ Res Sec A.* 1999;80:383-388.

10. Vom Saal FS, Hughes C. An extensive new literature concerning low-dose effects of bisphenol-A shows the need for a new risk assessment. *Environ Health Perspect.* 2005;113(8):926-933.

11. Osius N, et al. Exposure to polychlorinated biphenols and levels of thyroid hormones in children. *Environ Health Perspect.* 1999;107(10):843-849.

12. Soldin OP, O'Mara DM, Aschner M. Thyroid hormones and methylmercury toxicity. *Biol Trace Elem Res.* 2008;126(1-3):1-12.

13. Abdelouahab N. gender differences in the effects of organochlorines, mercury, and lead on thyroid hormone levels in lakeside communities of Quebec. *Environ Res.* 2008;107(3):380-392.

14. Cao Y, et al. Goitrogenic Anions, thyroid stimulating hormone, and thyroid hormone in infants. *Environ Health Perspect.* Online 2010;May 3rd.

15. Melzer D, et al. Association between serum perfluorooctanic acid and thyroid disease in the US national health and nutrition examination survey. *Environ Health Perspect.* Online 2010;Jan 20th.

Chapter IV

1. Barbosa Jr F, et al. A critical review of biomarkers used for monitoring human exposure to lead: advantages, limitations, and future needs. *Environ health Perspect.* 2005;113:1669-1674.
2. Frisch M, Schwartz BS. The pitfalls of hair analysis for toxicants in clinical practice: three case reports. *Environ Health Perspect.* 2002;110:433-436.
3. Partain RE, Drucker R, Fawcett J. EDTA suppositories for the removal of systemically toxic and cytotoxic heavy metals. *Townsend Letter.* 2007;287:128-132.
4. Crinnion WJ. The benefits of pre- and post-challenge urine heavy metal testing: Part 1. *Altern Med Rev.* 2009 Mar;14(1):3-8.
5. Crinnion W. Environmental medicine, part three: long-term effects of chronic low-dose mercury exposure. *Altern Med Review.* 2000;5(3):209-223.

Chapter V

Air

1. Rogers, S. *The E.I. Syndrome.* Prestige publ. Syracuse NY.
2. Hollender J, et al. *Naturally Clean.* New Society Publ. Gabroila Island, BC. Canada 2006.

Home

1. Hollender J, et al. *Naturally Clean.* New Society Publ. Gabroila Island, BC. Canada 2006.

2. Thomas, P. *What's in this stuff?* Penguin Group publ. NYNY. 2006.
3. Ladd DL. *Home Safe Home.* Tarcher Publ. 2005.
4. www.when.org.

Chapter VI

Mobilization

1. Jandacek RJ, Tso P. Enterohepatic circulation of organochlorine compounds: a site for nutritional intervention. *J Nutr Biochem.* 2007;18:163-167.
2. Jandacek RJ, et al. Effects of yo-yo diet, caloric restriction, and olestra on tissue distribution of hexachlorobenzene. *Am J Physiol Gastrointest Liver Physiol.* 2004;288:G292-G299.
3. Dahlgren J, et al. Persistent organic pollutants in 9/11 world trade center rescue workers: reduction following detoxification. *Chemosphere.* 2007:69(8):1320-1325.
4. Cecchini MA, et al. Chemical exposures at the world trade center. *Townsend Letter.* 2006;April:58-65.
5. Root DE, Katzin DB, Schnare DW. Diagnosis and treatment of patients presenting with subclinical signs and symptoms of exposure to chemicals which bioaccumulate in human tissue. Proceedings of the National Conference on Hazardous Wastes and Environmental emergencies. 1985;150-153.
6. http://www.detoxacademy.org/.
7. Zhao ZY, et al. The role of modified citrus pectin as an effective chelator of lead in children hospitalized with toxic lead levels. *Altern Therapies.* 2008;14(4):32-38.
8. Pande M, et al. Combined administration of a chelating agent and an antioxidant in the prevention and treatment of acute lead intoxication in rats. *Environ Toxicol Pharmacol.* 2001;9:173-184.
9. Wispritono B, et al. protection from cadmium cytotoxicity by n-acetylcysteine in LLC-PK1 cells. *J Pharmacol Exp Therap.* 1998;287(1):344-351.

10. Kalia K, Flora SJS. Strategies for safe and effective therapeutic measures for chronic arsenic and lead poisoning. *J Occup Health.* 2005;47:1-21.

11. Patrick, L. Toxic metals and antioxidants: part II: The role of antioxidants in arsenic and cadmium toxicity. *Altern Med Rev.* 2003;8(2):106-128.

Liver Detoxifcation

1. Nick, GL. Detoxification properties of low-dose phytochemical complexes found within select vegetables. *JANA* 2002;5(4):34-44.

2. Liska DJ, Bland J. Emerging clinical science of bi-functional support for detoxification. *The Townsend Letter.* 2002 October.

Detoxification Cofactors

1. Czap K. ed Vitamin A. *Alt Med Rev* Thorne Publ 2002 monographs vol 1:448-454.

2. Linninger S, et al. *The Natural Pharmacy.* Prima Health Publ. Rocklan, CA. 2nd ed 1999.

3. Czap K. ed Thiamine. *Alt Med Rev* Thorne publ 2002 monographs vol 1:416-420.

4. Jellin JM, et al. *Natural Medicines Comprehensive Database.* Therapeutic Research Foundation Publ. Stockton, CA 4th ed 2002.

5. Czap K. ed. Magnesium. *Alt Med Rev* Thorne publ 2002 monographs vol 1:251-260.

6. Nakachi K, et al. Influence of drinking green tea on breast cancer malignancy among Japanese patients. *Japan J Cancer Res* 1998;89:254-261.

7. Dulloo A, et al. Efficacy of green tea extract rich in catachin polyphenols and caffeine in increasing 24-hour energy expenditure and fat oxidation in humans. *Am J Clin Nutr* 1999;70:1040-1045.

8. Hall DC. Nutritional influences on estrogen metabolism. *Applied Nutr Science Reports.* 2001;1-7.
9. Marz RB. Medical Nutrition from Marz. Omni press. 2002.

Liver Cleansing Supplements

1. Linninger S, et al *The Natural Pharmacy.* Prima Health Publ. Rocklan, CA. 2nd ed 1999.
2. Mowrey DB. *The Scientific Validation of Herbal Medicine.* Keats Publ. New Canaan, CN 1986.
3. Murry MT. *The Healing Power of Herbs.* Prima Publ. Rocklan, CA. 2nd ed 1995.
4. Jellin JM, et al. *Natural Medicines Comprehensive Database.* Therapeutic Research Foundation Publ. Stockton, CA 4th ed 2002.
5. Gruenwald J, et al. *PDR for Herbal Medicines.* Medical Economics Co Publ. Montvale, NJ. 2000.
6. Liska DJ, Roundtree R. The role of detoxification in the prevention of chronic degenerative diseases. *Applied Nutritional Science report.* 2002.

Estrogen Detoxification Supplements

1. Higdon JV, et al. Cruciferous vegetables and human cancer risk: epidemiologic evidence and mechanistic basis. *Pharmacol Res.* 2007;55(3):224-236.
2. Rogan EG. The natural chemopreventive compound indole-3-carbinol: state of the science. *In Vivo.* 2006;20(2):221;228.
3. Head KA, ed. Calcium-D-Glucarate. *Alt Med Rev* 2002;7(4):336339.
4. Walaszek Z, Hanausek-Walaszek M, Webb TE. Antiproliferative effects of dietary glucarate on the Sprague-Dawley rat mammary gland. *Canc Lett.* 1990;49(1):51-57.
5. Patrick L. Toxic metals and antioxidants: part II. *Alt Med Rev* 2003;8(2):106-128.

6. Pande M, et al. Combined administration of a chelating agent and an antioxidant in the prevention and treatment of acute lead intoxication in rats. *Env Toxico Pharm* 2001;9:173-184.

7. Zahid M, et al. Inhibition of depurinating estrogen-DNA adduct formaiton by natural compunds. *Chem Res Toxicol.* 2007;20:1947-1953.

8. Flier J, et al. The neuroprotective antioxidant ALA induces detoxification enzymes in cultured astroglial cells. *Free Radic Res* 2002;36(6):695-699.

9. Hall DC. Nutritional influences on estrogen metabolism. *Applied Nutr Science Reports.* 2001;1-7.

10. Nishizawa Y, et al. Effects of methylcobalamin on the proliferation of androgen-sensitive or estrogen-sensitive malignant cells in culture and in vivo. *Int J Vitamin Res.* 1997;67(3):164-170.

11. Pietrzik k, Bailey L, Shane B. Folic acid and L-5-methyltetrahydrofilate: comparison of clinical pharmacokinetics and pharmocodynamics. *Clin Pharmacokinet.* 2010;49(8);535-548.

Let's Get It Out

1. Boyle, Wade, ND, and Saine, André, ND, *Lectures in Naturopathic Hydrotherapy*, (East Palastine, OH:Buckeye Naturopathic Press) 1988.

2. Gaginella TS, et al. Castor oil: New lessons from an ancient oil. Phytotherapy Res. 1998:12:S128-S130.

3. Grady H. Immunomodulation through castor oil packs. J Naturopathic Medicine. 1999;7(1):84-88.

4. Ishikawa T. The ATP-dependent glutathione S-conjugate export pump. *Trends Biochem Sci.* 199;17(11):463–468.

5. Richards DG, et al. Colonic Irrigations: A review of the historical controversy and the potential for adverse effects. *J Altern Compl Med.* 2006;12(4):389-393.

6. Walker M. Value of colon hydrotherapy verified by medical professionals prescribing it. *Townsend Letter.* 2000;205/206:66-71.

7. Briel JW, et al. Clinical value of colonic irrigation in patients with continence disturbances. *Dis Colon Rectum.* 1997;40(7):802-805.

8. Hildenbrand G. A coffee enema. *Healing Newsletter.* 1986;May-June.

9. Gerson, M. The cure of advanced cancer by diet therapy: a summary of 30 years of clinical experimentation. *Physiol Chemist and Physics.* 1979;10(5);449-464.

Glossary

1. Vom Saal FS, Hughes C. An extensive new literature concerning low-dose affects of bisphenol A shows the need for risk assessment. *Environ Health Perspect.*2005;113(8):926-933.

2. Moore, G. *Living with the Earth: Concepts in Environmental Medicine.* 2ed Lewis Publishers. Boca Raton, FL. 2002 Chapter 5.

3. Moore, G. *Living with the Earth: Concepts in Environmental Medicine.* 2ed Lewis Publishers. Boca Raton, FL. 2002 Chapter 10.

4. Adamson RH, Thorgeirsson UP. Carcinogens in foods: Heterocyclic amines and cancer and heart disease. *Advances in Experimental Medicine and Biology* 1995; 369:211-220.

5. Moore, G. *Living with the Earth: Concepts in Environmental Medicine.* 2ed Lewis Publishers. Boca Raton, FL. 2002 Chapter 5.

6. Mendez MA, Arab, L. Organochlorine compounds and breast cancer risk. *Pure Appl. Chem.* 2003;75(11-12):1973-2012.

7. Pedersen s, et al. In vitro skin permeation and retention of parabens from cosmetic formulations. *Int J Cosmet Sci.* 2007;29(5):361-367.

8. Padungtod C, et al. Reproductive Hormone Profile among Pesticide Factory Workers. *JOEM* 1998; (40):1038-1047.

9. Cabello G, et al. A Rat Mammary Tumor Model Induced by the Organophosphorus Pesticides Parathion and Malathion, Possibly through Acetylcholinesterase Inhibition. *Environ Health Perspect* 2001;109(5): 471-478.

10. Gerhard I, et al. Pentachlorophenol Exposure in Women with Gynecological and Endocrine Dysfunction. *Environ Res Sec A* 1999:80:383-388.

11. Lovenkamp-Swan T, Davis BJ. Mechanisms of phthalate ester toxicity in the female reproductive system. *Environ Health Perspect.* 2003;111(2):139-145.

12. Crinnion W. Environmental medicine, Part 2-Health effects of and protection from ubiquitous airborne solvent exposure. *Altern Med Review* 2000;5(2):133-143.

INDEX

V

vegetables,   9, 10, 11, 16, 41, 44, 49,
        72, 102, 122, 131, 138, 157, 189,
        217, 218
Vitamin C,   78, 133, 135
vitamin D,   75, 76, 94
Vitamin E,   78, 118, 135
volatile organic compounds,   19, 24, 26,
        30, 57, 58, 106, 114, 196, 197

W

water,   14-24, 31, 32, 39- 41, 45, 48, 49,
        52, 54, 55, 60-63, 66-68, 70, 71,
        76, 83, 87-91, 95, 101, 104-109,
        115, 121, 122, 129, 131, 140-147,
        149-151, 156-158, 160, 166, 167,
        182, 184, 185, 187, 189-195, 197,
        203

X

xylene,   2, 21, 71, 110, 113, 196

Z

zinc,   57, 78, 130, 133, 136, 189, 209,
        212